NATURAL MIGRAINE RELIEF: A HOLISTIC APPROACH TO MANAGING MIGRAINE

-DR. ASHISH SRIVASTAVA

TABLE OF CONTENT

PREFACE

Migraines are far more than headaches. For millions of victims worldwide, they constitute a complex condition often accompanied by serious disabilities that is negatively affecting the course of daily life, production, and quality of life in general. There is a fear of uncertainty at the time of an attack, which may lead to missed workdays and scarred plans with loved ones and nagging questions of when the next attack may hit. It may even be like hell one can never get out from for chronic migraineurs, for instance.

I have come to learn, in the years of research and patient discussions with migraine patients, that relief comes in many different forms. Sometimes conventional medications work well but lose their effectiveness or cause side effects that may become primary complaints over time. There's a general integrated approach in terms of triggers being addressed, natural benefits provided, and working throughout life without people needing to find it.

The book is a science-based approach written for those who want to take control of their migraine management. It's written based on science, and what's assembled so far is synthesised from the latest in research and pooled from expertise by health practitioners combined with personal stories on living well with migraines. I want to share with you these insights in a way that's almost giving you tools and knowledge that could be applied right now.

Each chapter of this book covers a different aspect of migraine management, from dietary changes and supplements to lifestyle habits and environmental adjustments. You'll find tips on identifying triggers, building a migraine-friendly environment, and creating routines that support your body's natural resilience.

But nothing, really-this book keeps it so simple and uses the real-life application of the strategy. It simply puts each concept in straightforward language, where you can even discover relatable examples showing how these strategies work out in real life. So I have used illustrations to make the content really engaging and easy to digest.

Now, I will believe in natural strength, but I also know that people may have different journeys to embark on. That's not actually bypassing medical advice, but rather it is more of a companion that usually complements your healthcare plan. Always consult a healthcare provider so you are sure the methods you choose are safe and appropriate for your specific needs.

If you are ready to take over your migraines and explore the natural methods going alongside the rhythms of the body, then this book is for you. In any case, I hope it helps and brings you closer to a life where migraines do not prevent you.

INTRODUCTION

Migraines affect millions of people worldwide. Migraines affect all demographics, ages, and lifestyles. For many others, it is more than sometimes being endowed with occasional headaches; it is a chronic condition that adversely affects quality life. The intensity and unpredictability of symptoms make it hard for other people to fully grasp what those who suffer go through.

This is true because during such emergencies, people largely rely on medications for only a temporary relief, and over time drawbacks are associated with the medication, one of which may be side effects, cost, and dependency.

Imagine being able to reduce, or even avoid, migraines. Imagine just going about your day without being held hostage by the anxiety of acute pain or any reliance on medication. This book is your journey through all of the non-medical ways to treat and prevent migraines, giving you tools for a life less painful.

WHY TREAT NATURE FOR MIGRAINE RELIEF?

This natural approach simply makes sense-for it treats the body as an entity, not just the symptoms that present themselves but gets at underlying causes, offering a more sustainable route toward wellness. This medical approach does not just insist on eliminating symptoms but rather seeks to prevent migraines by focusing on triggers and imbalances in the body.

For many, chronic migraines have something to do with the everyday aspects of life that they can control, such as diet, sleep, stress, exercise, and environmental elements. What's beautiful about natural migraine relief is that it empowers you: you're not fated to suffer at the whims of a migraine, but rather, you get steps for understanding and managing the factors that might be driving your migraine attacks.

A FRAMEWORK FOR QUALITY, EVIDENCE-BASED ANSWERS

Every chapter is meant to guide you step-by-step through a different aspect of natural migraine relief, supported by credible research as well as real-life examples and practical tips. Each remedy, practice, or lifestyle change discussed here has been chosen based on scientific evidence as well as from experiences of those who have benefited from these methods.

A HOW-TO GUIDE, NOT A SILVER BULLET

Realistic Expectations: Natural remedies take time. Remedies in this book are not to be used for overnight fixes, but rather for practical and sustainable reductions in the strength and occurrence of migraines over the long term. More often than medicine, therapies in this book focus on resilience and balance rather than fixation on a quick fix, which in contrast could offer instant relief without much attention being paid to the real causes. You'll find some methods work better than others for you, and that's perfectly fine. There is a winning method for everyone's lifestyle and body chemistry. The purpose of this book is to give you options and provide you with information so you can make informed choices. And every chapter is built so that you can customise the plan to exactly fit your needs, so you'll create a personal toolkit for migraine relief. Let's start this journey to headache-free living. Remember as you read through each of the chapters, the millions of other people who have now learned how to manage and get out of migraines naturally. You belong to a community of like-minded people seeking improvement in health and freedom from pain. The journey is long; still, the rewards run deep, and the journey is well worthwhile. With this guide in hand, you'll discover that migraine management is more than just treatment; it's a pathway to a healthier, balanced, and pain-free life. So, let's dive in and take the first step towards achieving headache-free living.

CHAPTER 1: UNDERSTANDING MIGRAINES

Migraines are complex neurological events, often misunderstood and sometimes dismissed as "just headaches." However, anyone who has experienced a migraine knows that it's a different kind of pain entirely—one that can disrupt work, social activities, and even basic daily functioning. To effectively manage migraines, it's essential to understand what they are, the types of migraines, common triggers, and the phases that many sufferers go through.

WHAT IS A MIGRAINE?

A migraine is more than just head pain; it's a recurring neurological condition marked by intense, throbbing pain, usually on one side of the head. Migraines are often accompanied by other symptoms, such as nausea, vomiting, and extreme sensitivity to light, sound, and smell. They can last anywhere from a few hours to several days, making them a serious disruption to daily life.

Migraines affect people differently. Some people may experience migraines only a few times a year, while others suffer from them several times a month. The unpredictability of migraines adds to the frustration, as sufferers often don't know when an attack might strike.

WHY DO MIGRAINES HAPPEN?

The exact cause of migraines isn't fully understood, but research suggests that they're related to abnormal brain activity that affects nerve signals, chemicals, and blood vessels in the brain. This abnormal activity can be triggered by various factors, from stress to hormonal changes and even certain foods.

While the brain doesn't have pain receptors, it's surrounded by blood vessels, meninges (brain linings), and nerves that can produce pain when stimulated. During a migraine, scientists believe that certain brain cells become overactive, causing the release of chemicals like serotonin, which narrow blood vessels and create a sensation of intense throbbing.

TYPES OF MIGRAINES

Understanding the type of migraine you experience can be helpful in managing it. There are several kinds, each with distinct characteristics:

1. Migraine Without Aura

This is the most common type of migraine, typically characterised by intense throbbing on one side of the head, nausea, and sensitivity to light and sound. These migraines don't include a warning "aura" phase but can last anywhere from four to 72 hours.

2. Migraine With Aura

About 25% of people with migraines experience an aura. An aura is a group of sensory disturbances that appear before the headache phase. Symptoms may include visual changes (like seeing zigzag lines or flashing lights), tingling sensations, or difficulty speaking. Aura typically lasts for 20–60 minutes before the headache begins.

3. Chronic Migraine

This type of migraine is defined by the frequency of attacks, occurring on 15 or more days per month for at least three months. Chronic migraines can include both headache days and symptom-free days, making it a particularly challenging form to manage.

4. Hemiplegic Migraine

A rare type, hemiplegic migraines cause temporary weakness or paralysis on one side of the body, similar to a stroke. Symptoms may also include visual disturbances and speech issues. Although frightening, the symptoms usually resolve after the migraine.

5. Menstrual Migraine

Many women experience migraines related to hormonal changes around their menstrual cycle. Menstrual migraines usually occur just before or during menstruation, when oestrogen levels drop.

6. Vestibular Migraine

This type of migraine includes dizziness, balance issues, and vertigo, often without a significant headache. People with vestibular migraines may experience nausea and a sensation of motion even while sitting still.

7. Silent Migraine

Silent migraines involve the typical aura phase but without the headache pain. Symptoms might include visual disturbances, nausea, or light sensitivity.

PHASES OF A MIGRAINE

Migraines typically come with a discernible set of patterns or phases. Once you know what these stages are, you can quickly recognize a migraine and control it before things get out of hand.

1. Prodromal Stage

This prodrome phase would be more of a form of "alert warning" that may begin anywhere from several hours up to even a few days before the attack totally sets in. Some patients experience changes in mood, food cravings, neck stiffness, greater than usual thirst or urination, and excessive yawning. The sufferer can thus prepare for an attack with such minor symptoms.

2. Aura Phase

Not all migraines have an aura, but for those that do, it is usually a big sign that the migraine is on its way. People who have an aura may see blinded spots or flashes of lights in their visual field, can become hard of speech, undergo numbness or tingling on the face or hands, and even develop temporary loss of eyesight. The aura always lasts less than one hour, and the headache usually starts before the aura ends.

3. Headache phase

Headache is the primary symptom associated with this stage, which is of high intensities of pulsating nature, unilateral and can be moderate to very severe in severity and aggravated by physical activity. In addition to headache, nausea and vomiting, photophobia, phonophobia, and hyperosmia occur during this stage. This stage can last between a few hours and three days.

4. Post-ruminal Phase

Most people fall victim to a postdrome phase, often referred to as a "migraine hangover," once the headache subsides. The postdrome phase involves lingering fatigue, mood changes, and feelings of general misery. Patients in the postdrome phase look drained, as well and are unable to concentrate for a day or so after the end of the migraine.

TRIGGERS: WHAT TRIGGERS A MIGRAINE?

Migraines are induced by diversity among different people; discovering what triggers yours can prevent such events from occurring. Here are some of the most common migraine triggers:

Stress: Emotional stress, anxiety, and tension are the major culprits behind migraine headaches. In stressful situations, your body releases some chemicals such as cortisol and adrenaline that precipitate a migraine.

Hormonal Changes: Especially in women, changes or fluctuations in oestrogen can cause and exacerbate migraines. Hormonal changes include those that occur during menstruation, pregnancy, and menopause.

Dietary Triggers: Some are sensitive to certain foods and drinks. These include alcohol, especially red wine, caffeine, aged cheeses, and processed foods with preservatives.

Sleep Disturbances: Both oversleeping and undersleeping can serve as migraine triggers. Consistency in sleep patterns is key in regulating the frequency of migraine attacks. Some might feel that changes in the barometric pressure, too much temperature, or high humidity are 'migraine triggers'. Bright or flickering lights, extremely strong odours such as perfume or smoke, and loud noises are the most common stimuli.

WHY KNOWING YOUR TRIGGERS MATTERS

Controlling a headache often starts with knowing what your specific triggers are. The tracking of symptoms and establishing patterns will have you better anticipating when an attack may strike, allowing you in certain instances to take actions which may head off an oncoming migraine. People will often keep a "migraine diary" of things they think somehow contributed to the attack, and through time, this can help them pattern something.

CONCLUSION

Migraines are complex neurological conditions that can come in very varied forms and severity. Knowing which types of migraines exist and the pattern of an attack can help in the better management of symptoms and appropriate forms of treatments. Identification and tracking of triggers can make you more empowered to cut down the frequency and intensity of migraine attacks.In the next chapter, we will look into what's often considered the intrinsic cause of migraines and how genetic makeup, chemical disposition of the brain, and other patterns of living can predispose someone to susceptibility to migraine headaches. With that knowledge you can begin your own journey toward a more self-empowering and natural approach to migraine relief.

CHAPTER 2: ROOT CAUSES OF MIGRAINES

Migraines don't happen by chance; they are complex nervous phenomena with deep biomedical, environmental, and lifestyle causes. For most patients with migraine, the attacks don't occur in isolation but are part of a recurrent attack pattern, possibly influenced by multiple triggers and contributing causes. This chapter will outline what may be causing your migraines-and how to cope with them naturally.

GENETIC FACTOR: IS MIGRAINE INHERITED?

Studies show that migraine has a strong genetic factor. In other words, if you have parents or siblings diagnosed with this condition, you are more likely to develop it too. There is as much as an 80% likelihood of hereditary factors being involved in the generation of migraines: clear evidence points to a predisposition in people who have them.

But genetics is not the entire story. Many genes can predispose people to migraine more, and lifestyle and environmental circumstances seem to be a big deal in triggering the episodes. It does not mean that even if you are genetically predisposed to migraines, you don't have a choice, and forever you have to remain a migraine sufferer. Understanding of your triggers and adoption of preventive measures will often control the frequency and severity of an attack, even if it runs in your family.

BRAIN CHEMISTRY ROLE IN MIGRAINE ATTACKS

Another specific cause of migraines is through the chemical processes in the brain, particularly with neurotransmitters. Neurotransmitters are chemicals that transmit signals in the brain between nerve cells. Migraine patients have, in their brain, imbalances in some neurotransmitters, such as serotonin and dopamine, which seem to act as triggers for migraine attacks.

Serotonin is one of the major neurotransmitter chemicals implicated in the pathogenesis of migraine. In the brain, serotonin's concentration fluctuates during an attack, leading to vasodilation and subsequent vasoconstriction in blood vessels; this would explain the throbbing pain, a hallmark of migraines. A gradual decline in serotonin concentration will cause it to follow some pathways that trigger pain; such a pathway leads to the events during an attack.

Dopamine is another major neurotransmitter. In some recent research, it's been discovered that altered levels of dopamine correlate with migraines. People become more sensitive to these trigger factors-bright lights, loud noises, and specific foods-following a shift in dopamine levels. Lifestyle adjustments and natural remedies have alleviated conditions for many sufferers by thwarting and normalising these neurotransmitters.

HORMONES AND MIGRAINES: THE ROLE OF OESTROGEN

Migraines in women are caused by a lot of hormonal fluctuations. Of women patients who experience migraines, up to 60 percent say that an attack is associated with the menstrual cycle, mainly caused by changes in oestrogen levels through the effects it has on how the brain maps it's pain pathways and can trigger the onset of an attack by suddenly diminishing.

This fluctuation in hormones is the reason why most women experience a migraine either before or even during their menstrual period, at which time the oestrogen level reaches its weakest point. Migraines may also be intensified during menopause or any phase of hormonal shift, such as pregnancy. Understanding these shifts can help you detect and prepare for migraine attacks. Monitoring the cycle and finding ways to balance hormones with natural means can keep hormone-related migraines to a minimum.

ENVIRONMENTAL AND LIFESTYLE TRIGGERS

Although genetics, brain chemistry, and hormones underlie the basic framework that predisposes a person to migraines, it is typically environmental and lifestyle triggers that bring on an attack. Here's a closer look at some of them:

Diet and Migraines

There are also specific foods and drinks that have been proven to cause migraine in some. Such examples include alcohol, aged cheeses, processed meats, foods, preservatives, or artificial additives.

Some have migraines due to consumption of foods that contain tyramine. Tyramine is an amino acid contained in aged cheese, smoked fish, and fermented food. Other suspected food triggers include artificial sweeteners aspartame. A food diary, therefore, can help you identify what and which of these food items are causing your migraine attacks so that you can make the required dietary changes.

Dehydration and Electrolyte Imbalance

This is probably the single most neglected trigger for migraine headaches. Low fluid volume can create electrolyte imbalances that irritate nerve function and create problems with blood flow. Some individuals have such sensitive heads that slight dehydration will precipitate a migraine. At-risk persons should drink high volumes of fluids, particularly in hot weather, and following and during exercise.

Sleep Patterns and Migraines

Probably the foremost causes of migraines are sleep disorders. Although oversleeping is somewhat related to migraine, it shifts the body's chemical equilibrium, whereby a lack of rest may provoke an attack. In these patients, abnormal sleeping may also become a weakness for most who suffer from migraines. For this reason, balancing your inner body clock can be enhanced by developing a regular sleeping pattern and a soothing bedtime environment.

Physical and Emotional Stress

Stress, both physical and emotional, also remains the most frequent precipitant as reported in most patients who experience migraines. Physical or emotional stress can cause hormonal secretions such as cortisol and adrenaline that do make a difference in the normal functioning of blood vessels and neurotransmitters. These changes directly trigger a migraine. Chronic stress will cause patients to have disrupted sleep, digestion, and immune systems, creating a vicious circle that exacerbates migraine. Coping mechanisms for stress should be useful as stress can make the headache more frequent and intense.

Meditation, exercise, or deep breathing techniques can reduce stress levels, subsequently increasing the number of triggers that can cause a migraine.

COMMON SENSORY TRIGGERS

Sensory Stimulation Bright or flashing lights, strong sounds, or pungent smells are some of the common sensory triggers that provoke a migraine. Such overstimulation triggers seem to overwhelm the brain of the hyper-responsive types. The percentage of migraines originating due to sensory triggers is very high, and the avoidance of over stimulating settings can make all the difference for someone with a migraine

VARIATIONS IN WEATHER AND ATMOSPHERIC PRESSURE

Changes in the weather are another easily adjusted trigger that can bring on migraines. Unfortunately we can't control the weather, but knowing how it affects migraines helps one plan around known precipitating factors. For instance, remaining indoors on extremely hot or humid days and gaining an environment with a consistent air conditioner for some can help regulate weather-related migraines.

WHY UNDERSTANDING ROOT CAUSES MATTERS

Knowing what triggers a migraine: knowing more than just the presence of information in your wallet; knowing what tools you have to make you strong enough to take control of your own health. This recognition of factors peculiar to you is step one in beginning to chart out a strategic way of preventing or managing attacks.

The Power of Awareness

It is the initial step that becomes very imperative-a sort of awareness. People who suffer from migraines do not realise just how much role their variable lifestyle contributes to their illness until unless they begin to track their symptoms as well as their lifestyle activities. The awareness generated can help you better in taking proper diet, sleep, stress-related lifestyle, and avoiding other triggers that cause migraine head-aches in the long run.

Managing Multiple Triggers

Migraines typically are multifactorial, that is, multiple causes. Maybe you have a tendency to the problem, but for you, certainly, stress and disturbances in sleep might be your greatest triggers that set off episodes. Often, treating each factor yields pretty significant improvements.

CONCLUSION:

Genetics and brain chemistry are the main sources of risk, but neither is likely to act alone; lifestyle and environmental factors greatly contribute to predisposition toward migraine.

One of the other most common things that trigger a migraine in the female gender is hormonal changes, especially estrogen. 3. Migraine frequency and severity may be impacted by diet, sleep, hydration, stress, and sensory trigger management. 4. Understanding the individual's specific triggers and underlying cause is essential for the development of an individualised, targeted approach to migraine prevention. In the following chapter, we will continue our discussion concerning dietary and hydration influences on the management of migraines. As you begin to learn how diet and hydration influences your chemistry and your health, you are going to make better choices for a potentially migraine-free lifestyle.

CHAPTER 3: THE ROLE OF DIET AND HYDRATION IN MIGRAINE MANAGEMENT

Food is not only fuel but also medicine—or, in some cases, a potential trigger for migraines. The link between diet and migraines has been well-documented, with certain foods, additives, and eating habits known to increase the likelihood of an attack. In this chapter, we'll explore how diet and hydration impact migraine health, highlight specific foods that tend to trigger migraines, and discuss dietary habits that can help stabilise brain function and prevent attacks.

IMPACT OF DIET ON MIGRAINES

Diet influences, in general, the body's chemistry-neurotransmitter levels and blood sugar balance-both of which have been implicated in the onset of migraine. For example, hypoglycemia or lowered blood sugar can precipitate an attack in some patients. Certain foods contain substances that influence activity in blood vessels or promote inflammation-all factors associated with a migraine.

Role of Neurotransmitters in Migraines

As discussed in Chapter 2, certain chemicals such as serotonin and dopamine are very associated with migraine development. However, some foods may build them while others destroy their balance. For example, an amino acid known as tryptophan is available in foods such as turkey, cheese, and nuts, which the body uses to create serotonin. Through including these tryptophan-rich foods into your diet, you will be prone to stabilising your serotonin levels, hence making one not so susceptible to experiencing migraines.

FOODS TO AVOID: COMMON MIGRAINE TRIGGERS

Though triggers vary from person to person, some foods are more likely than others to provoke migraines. If you're prone to migraines, it can be helpful to limit or avoid these common trigger foods and monitor how your body responds. Here are some of the most frequent dietary culprits:

1. Aged Cheeses: Tyramine is another amino acid found in aged cheeses, which has proved to increase blood pressure and can also initiate migraine attacks. High tyramine cheeses include blue cheese, cheddar, and Swiss.

2. Processed Meats: Many processed foods contain preservatives such as nitrates or nitrites that may increase your chances of suffering from a migraine. These preservatives include frankfurters, cold cuts, salami, and sausages.

3. Alcohol: primarily red wine Alcohol is one of the most common migraine triggers for many individuals. Red wine seems to be especially incendiary for most consumers. It is likely that tannins, histamines, and sulfites-all of which are found in small quantities in red wine-contribute to migraine attacks.

4. Chocolate: Chocolate itself contains certain substances such as caffeine and phenylethylamine, that could be a migraine trigger for some. Try to abstain from chocolate for some few weeks and monitor changes that occur.

5. Caffeine: Both anti-caffeine and anti-migrainous effects were found from caffeine. It would sometimes relieve headache symptoms in low doses, but high doses or withdrawal can easily provoke a migraine. Trying to find one's balance, for instance limiting oneself to no more than one small cup of coffee or tea a day may help.

6. Artificial Sweeteners: Aspartame and sucralose have been reported by various people as causing migraine. Such sugar substitutes tend to affect the brain. As such, they are predominantly found in diet sodas, sugar-free candies, and low-calorie foods.

7. **Foods high in Monosodium Glutamate (MSG)**: High content of MSG is that tastier flavour enhancer found in most processed foods and sometimes Asian food. It could be excitotoxic by overstimulating some of the nerve cells in some cases which may lead to migraines.

NUTRIENT-RICH FOODS HELP TO PREVENT MIGRAINES

Although some dietary elements trigger migraine attacks, others may be used to totally help prevent those attacks. Nutrient-rich whole foods provide the brain with nourishment while providing delicate neurotransmitter balancing and reducing inflammation. Among the best food groups for a diet that is conducive for preventing migraine, include:

1. Leafy Greens and Other Vegetables: Magnesium, a mineral that has been proven to decrease the frequency and severity of migraine attacks, can be found in leafy greens such as spinach, kale, and arugula. Some vegetables, such as sweet potatoes and carrots, offer antioxidants that combat inflammation caused by such a migraine.

2. Whole grains: such as oats, quinoa, and brown rice lead to slow glucose release into the blood, and it is always preventive to sudden rises and falls that always accompany blood sugar: sure to lead to a migraine. They also have B vitamins that are closely related to energy and cerebral functioning.

3. Nuts and Seeds: Nuts and seeds, such as almonds, pumpkin seeds, and chia seeds contain magnesium and healthy fatty acids. They may also help stabilise blood sugar and add an anti-inflammatory effect.

4. Lean Protein: Sources Consuming lean proteins such as chicken, fish, and legumes in your diet will help stabilise the blood sugar level. Pairing these with whole grains or veggies is a good combination. Fish, especially salmon and mackerel, contains omega-3 fatty acids that help combat inflammation.

5. Fresh Fruits: Fresh fruits have berries, apples, and oranges that contain antioxidants and fibre and can help to balance blood sugar and reduce inflammation in the body. Bananas are especially helpful because they have magnesium and are gentle on the stomach and soothing, which is good for a person who is nauseous from migraines.

6. Herbs and Spices: There are some herbs and spices that have anti-inflammatory properties. For instance, ginger relieves nausea and migraine, a common symptom. However, the curcumin in turmeric helps to bring down the inflammation within the brain and body.

HYDRATION: WHY IT MATTERS FOR MIGRAINE MANAGEMENT

Hydration is one of the important preventive aspects of migraine attacks. The electrolyte imbalance due to dehydration disrupts nerve function and blood flow within the brain in ways that predispose individuals to migraines. Here are a few hydration tips specifically for migraine sufferers:

1. Fluid Intake Consistently throughout the day: Encourage fluid intake to be done consistently throughout the day rather than a single take. Taking frequent small amounts of fluid prevents the imbalances of electrolytes and is not dehydrating.

2. Drink electrolytes containing fluids: Electrolytes like sodium, potassium, and magnesium charge nerve activity. Electrolyte-containing fluids such as coconut water, high in potassium, can be a godsend to keep hydration up. Do avoid products known as sports drinks that may boost your body's water uptake into your bloodstream, potentially boosting your blood sugar levels.

3. Restrict Diuretics: Drinks such as coffee, tea, and alcoholic beverages are diuretics because they stimulate urine production and can cause dehydration. If you're consuming these types of drinks, balance the intake with additional water.

4. Hydration through Foods: Hydration is also achieved through foods. Most fruits and vegetables contain a lot of water, thus aiding in hydration. Hydrating foods like watermelon, cucumbers, and oranges can be good additions to any diet aimed at preventing migraines.

MEAL TIMING AND BLOOD SUGAR STABILITY

Another very important factor in migraine prevention is maintaining steady blood sugar levels. Skipping meals, fasting or eating large ones infrequently can easily cause blood sugar fluctuations. Blood sugar fluctuation has been known to trigger migraines in some patients. Some tips on how to keep blood sugar levels stable are as follows:

Do not skip meals: Balanced meals ensure a constant sugar level within the body at all times. Maintain three balanced meals, and take a healthy snack if energy drops in the middle of the day.

Eat balanced food in meals: Each meal should have ideally all three components: protein, healthy fats, and complex carbohydrates. This combination delays digestion and determines the slow release of glucose through the bloodstream for long periods of time.

Consider Small, Frequent Meals: Some individuals find that having smaller meals more often-at about 3-4-hour intervals-can assist in avoiding blood sugar fluctuations. Healthy snack foods, such as a small portion of nuts or a piece of fruit, will be on hand.

KEEPING A FOOD AND MIGRAINE DIARY

One good tool for understanding what your personal migraine triggers might be is a food and migraine diary. Recording what you eat and drink, but noting how much it sparks migraine symptoms can help identify specific and patterns of triggers. Here's how to start:

1. Track all meals and snacks: Write down everything you eat and drink, as well as the time of day.

2. Track Your Migraine Symptoms: Record when the migraines occur, how intense they were, and what symptoms accompany them.

3. Look for Patterns: After a few weeks, take your diary and identify if there are specific foods or hydration-related triggers.

CONCLUSION

First of all, it is well noted that some foods, including aged cheeses, processed meats, alcohol, and caffeine are a common trigger for migraine headaches. Abstaining or reducing such foods may also prevent attacks.A diet rich in magnesium and antioxidants, with anti-inflammatory compounds, helps support brain function and reduce inflammation-both of which impact migraine prevention. Dehydration is a specific issue for many people who suffer from migraines. Consistent water intake, consumption of electrolyte-containing fluids, and use of fewer diuretics help keep dehydration from triggering migraines. Maintaining healthy blood sugar levels serves as an important management strategy for the migraines. Optimal blood sugar levels can be achieved by spreading meals well throughout the day such that fluctuations are avoided that may trigger the migraine attack. Maintaining a food and migraine diary may help you determine and avoid your specific dietary triggers. Dealing with Stress and Enhancing Sleep Lifestyle Interventions Needed Both can be crucial factors in the prevention of migraines. Knowing how the habits of your daily life affect your neurological health gives you control over proactive changes leading to fewer migraines and a life of better quality.

CHAPTER 4: STRESS MANAGEMENT AND SLEEPING SKILLS TO PREVENT MIGRAINE ENDS

Stress and sleep are the most crucial elements to be incorporated into the treatment of migraines. Both are known to be pretty strong contributors in terms of the frequency and severity of attacks. Chronic stress impacts brain chemistry, blood flow, and hormonal balance. Poor sleep also raises the sensitivity level of your brain to pain. You learn how to control stress and how to get quality sleep to make a lot of powerful, positive changes in yourself.

UNDERSTANDING THE CONNECTION BETWEEN STRESS AND MIGRAINE

Stress is another very common trigger for migraines. Stress can cause such a chain reaction in the body that will be manifested in an attack. When you are stressed, your body releases cortisol and adrenaline, which might temporarily affect levels of certain neurotransmitters or alter the blood vessel function. For a migraine sufferer, this disruption would initiate all too easily.

Chronic stress is especially problematic because it thrusts the body into a state of "fight or flight" that can persist for so long that chronic tension, fatigue, and sleep disturbance-all of which can make migraines worse-result.

Physical and Emotional Stressors

All stressors are not created equal, though, and all may impact migraine health. Here's a look at some common stressors and their potential effects:

1. Physical Stress: A type of physical stress is overexertion at some time when an individual may be working out or not getting enough rest that can increase tension in the muscles and disrupt blood flow that may lead to a migraine attack.

2. Emotional Stress: Emotional stress, for example, due to relationship conflicts, meeting work deadlines or financial stress, tends to affect hormone levels as well as neurotransmitter function. Chronic emotional stress generally leads to increased migraine frequency.

3. Environmental Stress: Conditions in a person's environment, such as noises or bright lights or an uncomfortable workspace, may be constant sources of stress that heighten susceptibility to migraines.

PRACTICAL TECHNIQUES FOR STRESS MANAGEMENT

While we cannot always escape stress, how we respond to it can mean the difference between triggering and controlling a migraine attack. Here are some easily practised techniques to reduce stress and keep your nervous system in balance:

1. Deep Breathing Techniques

Deep breathing stimulates the parasympathetic nervous system that is sometimes called the "rest and digest" state. Deep, slow breathing calms the nervous system, relaxes muscles, and lowers stress hormones. A few minutes of practice a day may alleviate stress levels.

How to Do It: Take a quiet spot for yourself and inhale through your nostrils for the count of four. Retain the breath for the count of four, then slowly exhale from your mouth for the count of six. Repeat this several times daily, or whenever you feel at increased stress.

2. Progressive Muscle Relaxation (PMR)

Another technique is progressive muscle relaxation, which would involve tensing and then relaxing of different muscle groups to release tension stored within the body. Many people go about their day with neck, shoulder, and jaw tension and that's basically what creates migraines. PMR might help loosen it up as well as induce relaxation.

How to Do It: Tense each muscular region (feet, calves, thighs, etc.) from your toes, holding for a few seconds then relaxing. Move up the body from there, tensing and relaxing at each area all the way up to the head. Pay special attention to areas that feel particularly tense.

3. Mindfulness Meditation

Mindfulness meditation teaches you the importance of being in the present moment. You have to step back from stress and not get derailed by anxious thoughts. Studies have also shown that mindfulness practice reduces migraine frequency and severity through regulation of stress responses and improvement in mood.

How to Do It: Spend 5-10 minutes each day in silent meditation. Sit in a relaxed way and with closed eyes. Focus on your breath. As soon as a thought enters your head, lightly note it and then refocus back to your breath.

4. Regular Physical Activity

Exercise Stress goes a long way in being reduced by exercise. Physical activity releases endorphins, which are natural mood elevators. Exercise helps boost your resilience to stress, so get moving. But steer clear of high-intensity exercise if that's what triggers your migraines. Try low-impact exercises like walking, swimming, or yoga. These activities are less likely to provoke a migraine.

5. Journaling

You can write down your thoughts and feelings to work them through. Writing down your worries, frustrations, or experiences may help you cope with emotional tension, so it has been seen as one method of reducing stress.

How to Do It: Take some minutes daily, or whenever you are feeling anxious, to write in a journal. You might spend your time writing about whatever stressors you are experiencing and things you are grateful for. The acts of gratitude have been shown to help people lower their levels of stress.

THE ROLE OF SLEEP IN CONTROLLING MIGRAINES

Good sleep is crucial for healthy brain usage, emotional endurance, and in preventing a migraine attack. If one does not get proper sleep, it generally lowers the pain threshold and makes the individual more sensitive to stimuli, thereby making them more susceptible to migraines. A consistent sleep pattern and a relaxing bed environment can work wonders for a migraine sufferer.

Poor Sleep as a Trigger of Migraine

This means that sleep causes the lack of restorative processes that the body should undergo within its deep sleep stages. This can disrupt brain activity and neurotransmitter levels, factors that may lead to increasing migraine attacks. Disrupted sleep habits can trigger an increase in cortisol levels, thereby enhancing the stress load on the body.

Create a sleep-friendly routine

This also creates a wake-sleep schedule that in turn continues to influence the stabilisation of your body's internal clock, thus making sleep easier and waking up more at regular times. Here are some key steps:

1. Go to bed and wake up at the same time every day: even on weekends. The constancy helps stabilise the body's internal clock and will bring about deeper, restorative sleep.

2. Make a Bedtime Pre-Sleep Ritual: Relaxing Creating a pre-sleep routine helps your body begin to associate that it's time for bed. It could be when you take a warm bath, read a book, or practise some relaxation exercises.

3. Avoid using screens in the bedroom or restrict screen time: At least an hour before bedtime because of the interference blue light from phones, tablets, and computers can have with melatonin production, the sleep hormone.

4. Sleep Environment: Try to make your bedroom cool, quiet, and dark. Blackout curtains, earplugs, or a white noise machine can help eliminate light or noise disturbances that may interfere with sleep.

5. Avoid Heavy Meals and Caffeine Before Bed: Heavy meals make you uncomfortable, and caffeine can hamper sleep. Try to have your last meal two hours before you go to bed at night and refrain from taking caffeine in the afternoon or evening.

NATURAL SUPPLEMENTS FOR STRESS AND SLEEP

There are several natural supplements that help with stress and excellent quality of sleep. These should only be taken under the guidance of a health care provider because of potential drug interactions.

Magnesium: This mineral is often referred to as the "relaxation mineral." It calms the nervous system, relaxing tension in the body. This can improve quality of sleep and reduce migraine frequency. Magnesium glycinate is a preparation best for inducing relaxation.

Melatonin: Melatonin is a hormone that controls sleep-wake cycles. Lower doses of melatonin can be taken 30 minutes before sleep to signal to your body that it's time to fall asleep, especially for those who often have difficulties falling asleep.

Valerian Root: Valerian root is one of the herbal supplements typically used to enhance relaxation as well as to improve sleep. The studies suggest it may reduce time to fall asleep as well as increase the quality of sleep.

Lavender: Lavender is known to promote relaxation; thus, will promote better sleep. You can use lavender essential oil in a diffuser or just add a few drops to your warm bath before bed.

TRACKING YOUR PROGRESS: A STRESS AND SLEEP DIARY

Keeping a diary of your stress levels, sleep patterns, and migraines can be very helpful in understanding the interactions of these factors. Through recording your everyday experiences, you may find specific patterns causing migraines and make appropriate changes.

Stress Log: Record moments of high stress every day, indicating common themes or triggers. Note down any stress-management techniques employed and rate their effectiveness.

Sleep Log: Record bedtime and wake-up time, and report your sleep quality night to night. Mark every disturbance, including waking in the middle of the night, and document any migraine symptoms you have at wake-up.

CONCLUSION

Stress represents one of the largest migraine triggers. Having an understanding of a person's stressors and educating him or her on how to relax by teaching relaxation techniques, such as deep breathing and mindfulness, reduces the trigger's effect. Good sleep hygiene is important for migraine management. Sleep routine can be developed by creating a bedroom that helps in relaxation and minimising its usages before sleep. Natural supplements such as magnesium, melatonin, and valerian root are sleep quality aids but always with a prescription from a health provider. Keeping a stress and sleep diary helps you identify patterns and allows you to make a claim about which of your stressors or sleep habits are contributing to your migraines. In the next chapter, we explore the role of exercise in managing migraines. Regular exercise improves the health of the brain, reduces stress, and stabilises hormones-all of which contribute to fewer and less severe migraines.

CHAPTER 5: THE ROLE OF PHYSICAL ACTIVITY IN MANAGING MIGRAINES

Exercise has many benefits toward health. For instance, it enhances the quality of heart health and moods. In addition, for people who suffer from migraines, specific benefits from exercise have been found: elimination of stress, an improvement in blood flow, and the automatic release of natural pain killers known as endorphins. Nevertheless, even though exercise could help prevent attacks, one needs to approach this a little bit sensitively since certain physical activities often provoke migraine attacks in particular individuals.

This chapter will illustrate the best exercise to patients suffering from migraines, creating a personal exercise plan, and preventing exercise-induced migraines.

HOW TO BENEFIT FROM EXERCISE IN MIGRAINE PREVENTION

Regular exercise has a myriad of effects on regulating several systems in the body, concerning migraines, including those that deal with the nervous system, circulatory system, and hormonal balance. Here's a rundown on how exercising prevents these:

1. Reducing Stress

Physical activities tend to reduce stress. Exercise aids in the release of chemicals whose effects on an individual's body may result in an improvement in mood. Some of these chemicals function as anti-anxiety and depression agents, thereby possibly lowering the overall level of stress. In Chapter 4, it was established that stress is one of the most common migraine triggers. Therefore, reducing stress due to physical activity may serve to reduce the frequency of migraines.

2. Improved Blood Flow

Circulatory exercise, for instance, increases circulation, which benefits the brain due to the presence of healthy blood flow. Since migraines are part and parcel of abnormal blood vessel functions, increased circulation tends to lower the chances of a migraine attack.

3. Increased Neurotransmitter Regulation:

The level of physical exercise determines the extent to which neurotransmitters like serotonin and dopamine are influenced. The chemicals play imperative roles in the control of mood swings and pain. The balancing of such neurotransmitters through exercise may create a well-balanced environment in the brain that is less susceptible to migraines.

4. Quality of Sleep:

Studies have shown that exercise improves quality of sleep by regulating the body's natural sleep-wake cycle. As we reviewed in Chapter 4, high-quality sleep is also known as migraine prevention. Regular exercise will enable you to sleep better.

5. Body Weight Regulation

Some people may have fewer migraine attacks when they are at a healthy weight. Having excess body weight is most likely to contribute to having an increased risk of developing migraines, especially for chronic migrants. Exercise encourages one to keep fit and in good weight. By taking care of one's weight, they will probably reduce the number of attacks they have due to this factor.

TYPES OF EXERCISE BENEFICIAL FOR MIGRAINE

Not all exercise is the same for a headache. High-intensity or high-impact exercise may indeed trigger an attack in a migraine sufferer. These are some of the good exercises for migraine patients:

1. Low-Intensity Aerobic Exercises

Low-impact aerobic exercises, such as walking, swimming, and cycling, can be tolerated by most people suffering from migraines. Such exercises enhance cardiovascular health without overstressing the body.

Walking: It is a gentle walk for 20-30 minutes to increase the blood flow, reduce stress, and induce relaxation. Walking outdoors can also bring with it fresh air as well as exposure to natural light, both of which are conducive to mood.

Swimming: Swimming is a great low-impact activity that provides much cardiovascular benefit with minimal joint strain. It can also be cool, so this can be a good option for those who are not hot-sensitive.

Cycling: Stationary or outdoor cycling at low to moderate pace is another good cardiovascular workout that doesn't have the high impact of running.

2. Yoga and Stretching

Yoga is particularly well suited to migraine patients because it integrates physical activity with the use of deep breathing and relaxation. The studies indicate that yoga helps decrease the frequencies and severity of migraines since an improvement in flexibility also lowers physical tension in the muscles as well as improves relaxation.

Yoga Benefits: It includes Improved flexibility, especially reduced muscle tension in the neck and shoulders; a clear calm mind space, which may help prevent migraine attacks; and this, along with breathwork, lays focus on relaxation and stress management.

Stretching: Regular stretching, especially for the neck, shoulders, and upper back, will start to untangle stress in areas that the migraine sufferer typically holds tension in. Getting a few of these stretches into your routine or as part of your cool-down after a workout will do the trick.

3. Tai Chi and Qigong

Tai Chi and Qigong are low-impact exercises that focus on slow, flowing movements, control of the breath, and mindfulness. These practices are extremely soft on the body and have well-known benefits for tension reduction, making them an excellent choice for persons suffering from migraines.

Benefits of Tai Chi and Qigong: Tai Chi and Qigong exercises help improve balance, flexibility, and mental acuity. While their movements are slow and controlled, they promote relaxation and enhance the flow of energy throughout the body, thus reducing the migraine frequency.

4. Strength Training - Moderation

Strength training at a moderate intensity may increase muscle tone, promote joint stability, and improve overall fitness--all potentially beneficial weight management effects for patients with weight-related migraine triggers.

Approach to Strength Training: Avoid heavy lifting or high-intensity resistance exercises because these exert a lot of tension on the muscles of the neck and head, which is a possible cause of migraine. Use moderate weight with more repetitions and allow sufficient time to master the form.

EXERCISE-INDUCED MIGRAINE AVOIDANCE

While exercise is mostly good, some activities or approaches may trigger migraines. Here are some strategies to help you enjoy the benefits of physical activity while minimising the risk of exercise-induced migraines:

1. Warm Up and Cool Down

Skipping a warm-up or cool-down can suddenly change the flow of blood and the muscle tension, which can cause a migraine. Warm up with some light movement for at least 5-10 minutes, for example by walking, before doing anything strenuous. Cool down with some flexibility exercises or easy movement to gradually bring your heart rate down.

2. Hydrate

One of the most common reasons for the occurrence of migraines is dehydration, especially if you had an intensive workout. Drink plenty of water before, during, and after your workout so you will be properly hydrated. If you are to exercise for longer periods, consider using electrolyte drinks to replace the minerals lost in your sweat.

3. Avoid Overheating

Overheating can trigger migraines; thus, avoid overheating during exercises. If you are exercising outdoors, adjust your exercise times into when it is coolest during the day. Wear light and airy clothes also. If you exercise indoors, ensure you have ventilation, and if need be, bring in a fan.

4. Monitoring the Intensity Level

Apart from migraine, intense exercise can cause common conditions in individuals but, in general, it can improve one's fitness. This is not to say that you must press your body to the extreme limit. Carefully monitor your intensity level during workout-mostly do light to moderate exercises; avoid high-intensity workout programs. So long as you feel dizziness, lightheadedness, or fatigue, it is proper to rest and sit calmly.

5. Maintain Good Posture

Especially if you tend to do some exercises incorrectly and are often lifting heavy weights during cycling, this will exert stress on your neck and head, thus causing you a migraine. Try to maintain the right posture and position while working out, and maybe enrol in classes with a trainer to ensure that you are doing the exercises correctly.

6. Listen to Your Body

The key rule of thumb is to listen to your body. When you sense that creeping, familiar pre-migraine feeling while exercising, stop right away. It also helps to know when one should rest. Overexertion and exercising when really low or under stress is more likely to lead to a migraine.

DESIGNING AN EXERCISE PLAN TAILORED TO YOUR NEEDS

An individualised workout plan based on the person's needs and tolerances is essential for physical activity as part of a migraine treatment program. Here is a model weekly schedule for a beginner below.

Day 1: 30 minutes of brisk walk + 10 minutes of stretching

Day 2: 20-30 minutes of yoga with emphasis on relaxation and breathing

Day 3: 20 minutes of light cycling or swimming

Day 4: Rest day or gentle stretches

Day 5: Tai Chi or Qigong for 30 minutes

Day 6: Strength training, light weights 20-30 minutes

Day 7: Rest

KEEPING AN EXERCISE AND MIGRAINE DIARY

By recording your exercises and migraine symptoms that coincide, you will start to identify what works best for you. Document each exercise, noting the following information:

Type and duration of exercise

i) Intensity
ii) Degree of hydration and any other activities undertaken, such as warm-up and cool-down
iii) Any symptoms that happen during or after exercise, such as dizziness, fatigue, or the onset of a migraine
iv) Review your diary in a few weeks and look for patterns or specific types of exercise that always seem to trigger a migraine. Adjust your plan based

on what you have found and focus on activities that seem to enhance the management of a migraine.

CONCLUSION

It is understood that physical exercise does indeed influence stress, blood circulation, and neurotransmitter regulation, all of which are beneficial to migraine prevention. However, this is relevant only in the context of the type of physical activity: it should be low in intensity with regard to the likelihood of inducing migraine. Low-intensity aerobic exercise - such as walking, swimming, or yoga - is probably the best for most people with migraine, in that it improves circulation without causing undue stress to the body while diminishing stress. Controlling exercise-induced migraines requires hydration, avoiding overheating, and listening to your body's signals. You may find that keeping an exercise and migraine diary will help you identify certain patterns of workout that make your headaches better or worse. From here, you can refine your approach over time.

In the following chapter, we will discuss how controlling other sensory triggers is important in trying to prevent a migraine. Light, sound, and other sensory factors cause changes in migraine frequency and severity.

CHAPTER 6: MANAGING SENSORY TRIGGERS TO PREVENT MIGRAINES

For most patients, sensory stimuli play a great major role in triggering attacks from migraines. Things such as certain lights or even smells trigger a patient very powerfully in the ways that result in symptoms of migraine. Understanding such triggers and managing them is one excellent way to decrease the frequency and severity of episodes caused by this migraine.

This chapter addresses the different types of sensory triggers, why such triggers might impact a migraine sufferer, and how such sensitivity might be managed in various environmental contexts.

Consumers who suffer from migraines also have something referred to as heightened sensory sensitivity, meaning that their brains are more sensitive to sensory input than those people who do not have migraines. In fact, the research is indicating that people who are afflicted with migraines may have overactive pain-processing centres within the brain, hence making them more sensitive to discomfort and triggering from certain sensory stimuli.

Here is a breakdown of common sensory triggers and how they can influence migraines:

1. Light Sensitivity (Photophobia)

Many patients are sensitive to light, especially bright or flickering. Fluorescent lights, the sun, and glare from screens often cause headaches. According to studies, overstimulation of the brain happens by light sensitivity which further triggers or worsens the migraine.

2. Sensitivity to Sound (Phonophobia)

People with migraines tend to find loud noises or sudden sounds extremely discomforting. Routine environmental triggers include loud music, construction noise, and crowded places. Many migraine sufferers also state that their sensitivity to smells tends to increase during the attack, causing much distress in itself.

3. Sensitivity to Smells (Osmophobia)

Other causes include strong smells such as perfumes, gasoline, or cleaning chemicals. Such odours can stimulate nerve pathways involved in the migraine process, especially in sensitive individuals.

4. Sensitivity to weather and environment

The changes in barometric pressure, humidity, and temperature can also trigger a migraine in certain people. Any such environmental changes may alter the blood flow and nerve sensitivity and make the brain more susceptible to migraine attacks.

LIGHT SENSITIVITY MANAGEMENT

Light sensitivity is one of the most common sensory triggers for migraines. Thus, some simple measures that would reduce bright or flickering light exposure would prevent an attack in the first place. Some practical ways to manage light sensitivity are as follows:

1. Lighting That Is a Migraine Friendly

Fluorescent lighting and other harsh artificial lights often act as a trigger for people with migraines. LED bulbs can be replaced with these lights or softer lighting used to produce more of a migraine-friendly environment.

Confer workstations near windows during the daytime to benefit from natural and filtered light instead of artificial light, for natural light is generally less harsh and soothing.

Dimmer Switches and Soft Lamps: This usually allows the installation of dimmer switches, which can be turned on and off according to mood, enabling you to darken the lights when you do not want to use bright lights. Soft lamps or indirect light (light reflected from walls rather than direct lighting) often reduces glare and eye strain.

2. Wear Tinted Glasses

Specialised tinted glasses can block wavelengths of light known to trigger migraines, particularly blue and green light. Studies show that some tints-even FL-41 lenses-have relieved light sensitivity in migraine sufferers.

Who to Wear Them and When: Wearing them indoors under fluorescent lights, outside when the sun is shining bright, or in front of your computer may be helpful. Most people find them beneficial when having an attack or at times they know they will be exposed to bright lights.

3. Restrict Screen Time and Employ Screen Filters

Computer and phone screens emit blue light, which is the cause of migraines in people. Restrict your screen time and make use of screen filters to reduce the effects of sensitivity to light.

Blue Light Filters: All devices offer a blue light filter setting that decreases the total emission of blue light. These are commonly known as "Night Shift" or "Comfort View" and can be set to go into effect automatically at night.

Breaks and Blinking: Pay attention to the 20-20-20 rule-watch something 20 feet away for 20 seconds every 20 minutes. This easily reduces eye strain in addition to potential screen-related migraine triggers.

4. Blackout Curtains and Sunglasses

If light-based triggers cause migraines, blackout curtains can definitely prevent bright sunlight at home. Sunglasses with polarised lenses also reduce glare while outdoors.

Polarised Sunglasses: If you have mild sensitivity to light, polarised sunglasses will minimise glare from reflective surfaces like water or car hoods.

STRATEGIES FOR MANAGING SOUND SENSITIVITY

In noisy settings, sound sensitivity may be a significant challenge for migraine patients to tackle their daily activities. Here's how to reduce the effects of sound on migraines:

1. Earplugs or Noise-Cancelling Headphones

Earplugs and noise-cancelling headphones have really become useful tools in sound management for those with high sensitivity to noise. These help them by reducing the impact of such sounds that could trigger their migraines.

Foam Earplugs: Foam earplugs cost little and are portable. They can be used in noisy rooms or even in bed when nighttime noises cause problems.

Noise-Cancelling Headphones: These are ideal for people who have a job or drive to work in a noisy traffic environment. Noise-cancelling headphones will mask noise to help prevent migraine headaches.

2. Have a Quiet Space

An escape haven from migraine-eliciting sounds can be created in a quiet room in the home or workplace. Make sure that sources of loud electronics and other noises are absent from the room.

White Noise Machines: White noise machines or apps can be used to provide an unchanging soft sound that can mask others. White noise might be just as effective when background noise is an unwinnable battle.

Sometimes, you need to get away from noisy situations. If you are in a crowded or noisy place, take a few minutes stepping outside or getting to a quieter place. Some short periods of quiet can prevent sensory overload and minimise the chance of getting a migraine.

SMELL SENSITIVITY CONTROL TECHNIQUES

Some smells are quite potent for triggering a migraine, and some of them are impossible to avoid. Here is how you can control smell sensitivity effectively:

1. Detect and Steer Clear of Harming Smells

Some people experience that some odours, for example perfume or cigarette smoke, seem to trigger migraines. Often, however, people find that other chemical or sweet smells are problems. By figuring out what smells trigger your symptoms, you can avoid these substances.

Odour-Free Products: Opt for fragrance-free products whenever available. This encompasses cleaning supplies, personal care items, as well as laundry detergents. Most any place sells a line of fragrance-free products.

Avoid Triggers: Avoid smelly grocery stores and markets, malls, tobacco aisles, and snack food aisles.

2. Essential Oils in Moderation

Some smells calm others stimulate the head, which can aid in the treatment of migraines. Research studies have found that lavender and peppermint oils will reduce migraine pain, but essential oils do trigger in some people.

Application Instructions: Try applying a few drops of a highly diluted essential oil to your temples or to your wrist, or diffuse a few drops. Be careful with any new scent for you to avoid using it as a trigger.

3. Good Ventilation

Good ventilation will also minimise the impact of pungent odours present in your environment. Keep your windows open or use an air purifier to allow air circulation within your house. This might help prevent smells from lingering and building within your home.

MANAGING WEATHER-RELATED TRIGGERS

The changing weather, especially the pressure barometer, may be a significant trigger for migraine attacks. You cannot exercise control over the changing conditions; however, here are some ways through which you might manage the changing weather impacts on your migraine condition:

1. Monitor the Changes in Weather

Tracking weather forecasts can help you anticipate what might trigger your attacks. For many patients, various apps or tools for tracking the weather can assist in anticipating attacks.

Apps tracking with migraine: There exist some apps that track your migraine, where you record your symptoms after which you correlate them with changes in the weather. This can finally help you to realise patterns that you will be able to head off by preventing such weather conditions.

2. Change Your Environment

If you are aware of some of the triggers like high humidity that cause migraines, then change your indoor atmosphere. This may include using a dehumidifier in humid weather or an air purifier when there is poor air quality to minimise the chances of having a migraine attack.

3. Prepare Advance

If you can predict weather changes, plan your day based on that. You may want to limit yourself from doing heavy activities, shorten your outdoor time, or have plenty of rest and tranquillity to allow your body to condition itself to the changes.

CONCLUSION

Determine what sensory stimulus triggers your migraines-for example, light sensitivity, noise sensitivity, specific odours, or changes in the weather.

Manage light sensitivity by wearing tinted glasses, limiting as much screen time as possible, and using soft lighting in the home and workplace.

Use noise-cancelling headphones or earplugs when outdoors to reduce sensitivity to sound.

Avoid smells by choosing fragrance-free products and good air ventilation in the home. Experiment with calming scents like lavender if they do not trigger migraines.

Follow the weather and make lifestyle changes if such patterns are contributing to a migraine attack.

In the following chapter, we will discuss dietary triggers and sensitivity as it relates to migraines. Certain foods and beverages are migraine triggers; therefore, knowing what makes you sensitive may help prevent a migraine attack.

CHAPTER 7: DIETARY TRIGGERS AND FOOD SENSITIVITIES

Diet is the biggest push in migraine management for most people. There are some foods and beverages laden with chemical substances that can cause migraine attacks. Some individuals' recurring migraines might be caused mostly by certain food sensitivities. As you learn about diet-migraine interplays and your particular food triggers, you'll find that you can make smart dietary choices to foster a headache-free lifestyle.

This chapter will take a closer look at common dietary triggers, the science behind them, and practical strategies for identifying and managing food sensitivities.

WHY SOME FOODS TRIGGER MIGRAINES

There are a number of reasons why food can trigger a migraine. Here's a look at some of the main factors:

1. Chemical Compounds in Food

Some foods contain chemical compounds known to influence the brain and blood vessels. Foods rich in tyramine, histamine, and nitrates may cause fluctuations in blood flow and altered neurotransmitter levels, which may trigger a migraine.

2-Blood Sugar Fluctuations

Other notable triggers include fluctuations in blood sugar, such as associated with skipping meals or gobbling down sugar, which cause headaches. Hypoglycemia, low blood sugar, has been reported to be a migraine trigger, and individuals who do not eat for long hours or eat high-sugar foods may be more prone to this.

3. Food Allergies and Intolerances

For instance, an allergy or intolerance to a specific food-such as dairy or gluten-will cause an inflammatory reaction, which is the reason for a migraine. Of course, no one would suggest that all migraine patients have food sensitivities.

However, when they do, there is the significant lessening of symptoms when said foods are excluded.

4. Caffeine Dependence and Withdrawal

Caffeine generally has a complex relationship with migraines. While some individuals find that small quantities of caffeine alleviate migraine for them, other people may experience migraines caused either by excessive use of caffeine or by abrupt caffeine withdrawal. General guidelines about intake can help avoid these peaks and troughs in controlling migraines.

5. Dehydration

Although not an actual food, dehydration is a common trigger; maintaining good hydration is one of the basic principles of prevention. Caffeinated or alcoholic drinks are diuretics, and hence can lead to dehydration.

COMMON MIGRAINE TRIGGER FOODS AND BEVERAGES

Trigger foods and beverages differ for every individual, yet several common triggers exist because of the following food and drinks:

1. Aged Cheeses

Tyramine is a chemical that is highly concentrated in aged cheeses, such as cheddar, blue cheese, and Swiss. It is widely recognized to produce an effect on blood pressure, and in individuals who are sensitive to it, the substance can provoke the start of a migraine attack.

2. Processed Meats

Processed meat products like hot dogs, bacon, sausage, and deli meats often contain nitrates or nitrites as preservatives. These agents would cause dilation of the blood vessels, which may initiate attacks of migraine.

3. Alcohol

Other people often complain that alcoholic drinks stimulate migraine attacks. Some of these drinks are red wine, beer, and champagne. These drinks contain histamines and sulfites, which contribute to headaches. Alcohol leads to dehydration, and this contributes to the risk of getting migraines.

4. Chocolate

Chocolate is a product containing caffeine and a compound named phenylethylamine, which may influence blood in the brain and be a natural migraine trigger to others.

5. Caffeine

However, excessive intake or sudden abstinence from caffeine is known to provoke the attack. It is recommended that one consume the same amount of caffeine daily and avoid excess consumption.

6. Artificial Sweeteners

Artificial sweeteners, primarily aspartame, are available in diet sodas, sugar-free foods, and some processed snacks. Some studies suggest that aspartame has an effect on neurotransmitters and often leads to more frequent migraine attacks in susceptible individuals.

7. MSG (Monosodium Glutamate)

MSG is a flavour enhancer found in many processed foods. Migraine sufferers relate MSG as the cause of their migraines, but no concrete evidence is found to link MSG to migraine headaches.

MSG is a flavour enhancer widely used in nearly all packaged foods, canned soups, and some Chinese dishes. Some people believe that this chemical causes them headaches and migraine attacks.

8. Salty and Highly Processed Food

Excessively processed foods with high sodium content are thought to cause an increase in blood pressure and activate the dehydration process in your body, which triggers migraine headaches.

KNOWING YOUR SPECIFIC DIETARY TRIGGERS

Since each person's triggers are different, there is usually a trial-by-error process in identifying food triggers. Here is a step-by-step approach to finding your own food sensitivities:

1. Food and Migraine Diary

A food diary will enable you to track what you take and whether it triggers any corresponding migraine symptoms. Record every meal, including the time and ingredients used, besides beverages you take. Note the duration when you get your migraine and what food might be triggering it, about that time.

What to Track: Note not just what you ate but when you ate it. Sometimes the timing really, really does make a difference. For instance, some foods may trigger a migraine within hours, and others within a day or two.

2. Try an Elimination Diet

An elimination diet is the removal of common trigger foods from your diet for a fixed period- typically two to four weeks-and then reintroducing them one by one and observing whether there are any adverse reactions.

Detailed Process:

Begin with the elimination of common migraine trigger foods including aged cheeses, processed meats, caffeine, and alcohol.

After a week or two, reintroduce one food at a time and see whether they provoke any symptoms of migraine.

If there is a food item that is commonly linked with an onset of a migraine, then it might simply be purged from the diet.

3. Consulting a Nutritionist or Healthcare Provider

The process of determining dietary triggers is much easier when following the orders of a nutritionist or healthcare provider. They can assist in leading through all the steps of the elimination diet, discuss healthy choices with rich nutrients, and make sure the changes in diet do not induce nutrient deficiencies.

REGULATION OF BLOOD SUGAR LEVELS TO PREVENT MIGRAINE

One of the key migraine prevention measures is steady blood sugar, especially if you suffer from low blood sugar. Here are some ways to keep your blood sugar steady:

1. Eat Regularly

One of the most obvious ways that skipping meals or going too long without eating can prevent blood sugar levels from stabilising is a common migraine trigger. Consume balanced meals every three to four hours to keep the blood sugar steady.

2. Balance carbohydrates with protein and healthy fats

Carbohydrates, which come from sugary snacks, can cause your blood sugar to shoot up and then plummet. Combining carbohydrates with protein and healthy fats, such as nuts, seeds, or lean meats, will slow digestion and maintain energy levels better while preventing swings in blood sugar.

3. Steer clear of high-sugar foods and drinks

Foods and beverages high in added sugar can cause blood sugar to spike and fall rapidly. Opt for whole, unprocessed foods like fruits, vegetables, and whole grains, which provide a steadier source of energy.

MANAGING CAFFEINE INTAKE

If caffeine is a trigger for you, consider moderating your intake to prevent caffeine-related migraines. Here are some guidelines:

Reduce Total Intake: Limit the total amount of caffeine to less than 200 mg daily, or around one to two cups of coffee. High levels of caffeine increase the likelihood of withdrawal headaches.

Stick to a Routine Pattern: Some individuals react to sudden changes in the amount of caffeine they consume. Quit caffeine slowly if you decide to stop it, and replace it with herbal teas or decaf beverages instead.

Hydrate: Because caffeine acts as a diuretic, staying hydrated by drinking plenty of water throughout the day can help neutralise its dehydrating effects and migraine risk.

CONCLUSION

Food triggers are often idiosyncratic to each individual, so a food and migraine diary can help identify your specific food sensitivities.

Common foods known to trigger a migraine can include aged cheeses, processed meats, alcohol, chocolate, caffeine, and foods containing artificial sweeteners or MSG.

Keep blood glucose levels in the normal range by regularly taking in nutritionally balanced meals in a constant and stabilised manner to prevent having a low blood glucose migraine. Consume caffeine in limited quantities and maintain usage at a consistent and controlled level. Drink plenty of fluids.

For an elimination diet, see a registered dietitian or your healthcare provider for guidance on how to follow this structured step-by-step process for determining your triggers.

In the following chapter, we will also talk about hydration and electrolyte balance in terms of prevention of migraines. Maintaining optimal hydration is important in migraine prevention, and understanding the relationship among dehydration, electrolytes, and migraines can be a powerful tool for reducing symptoms.

CHAPTER 8: HYDRATION AND ELECTROLYTE BALANCE FOR MIGRAINE PREVENTION

Our bodies are composed of large amounts of water, participating with every functioning of our body, from the transport of nutrients to regulating our body's temperature. For migraineurs, proper hydration is even more important since dehydration can be a powerful trigger for migraine. In fact, research studies revealed that even slight dehydration leads to headaches that can readily transform into full-fledged migraine attacks in predisposed persons.

This chapter aims to address why hydration is very important for migraine patients, where electrolytes play a role in the prevention of migraine, and practical ways on how one can stay hydrated while maintaining the balance of such ions in his body.

WHY HYDRATION IS VERY IMPORTANT IN PREVENTING MIGRAINES

Dehydration interrupts the balance of essential minerals in the body, which then causes a domino effect of physical responses culminating into headaches and migraines. Here's how it works:

1. Decreased blood circulation to the brain

Through dehydration, it reduces the volume of the blood; hence, it strains the flow of oxygen-rich blood to the brain. The brain is very sensitive to a change in oxygen levels, and low blood flow can cause headache symptoms.

2. Blood Pressure Level

It tries to compensate the body through retained water when one gets dehydrated, which enhances the blood pressure level. Such a change can work as a trigger among people prone to migraines.

3. Chemical Imbalance

Inadequate hydration can cause alterations in the levels of neurotransmitters in the brain, such as serotonin, which is responsible for pain modulation and mood control. Altered levels of serotonin have been associated with migraine attacks.

4. Higher susceptibility to other triggers

Dehydration causes increased susceptibility to other external migraine triggers like stress, lack of proper sleep, or irritation from some sensory stimulus because it leaves both the brain and body susceptible to these stimuli.

ROLE OF ELECTROLYTES IN HYDRATION AND MIGRAINE PROPHYLAXIS

While talking of hydration, most people only think of it in terms of water. Although, to maintain the hydration of the body, electrolytes have to come into the play - major minerals such as sodium, potassium, calcium, and magnesium. These minerals enable the balanced fluids that flow in and out of the cells, carry nerve impulses, and control muscle contractions, all crucial functions that help to keep these debilitating headaches away.

Some major electrolytes and their association with migraines:

1. Sodium

Na is essential for fluid balance, particularly in blood-filled vessels. Either too much or too little can cause fluctuations in blood pressure and may act as a migraine trigger in those who are sensitive to those changes.

2. Potassium

The presence of K promotes fluid balance, the contraction of muscles, and nerve impulses. Low potassium depletion will amplify the symptoms of dehydration and a risk of migraine attack.

3. Calcium

Calcium plays an important role in nerve signalling and muscle activity. When calcium is deficient spasm and headache result, and this probably contributes to the pain of migraine.

4. Magnesium

Magnesium plays a crucial role for patients suffering from migraine. More than 300 biochemical reactions are magnesium dependent and include relaxation of muscles and functioning of nerves. This level is very low in most patients with migraine, and magnesium supplementation helps decrease frequency and intensity of their migraine attacks.

SIGNS OF DEHYDRATION AND ELECTROLYTE IMBALANCE

Some knowledge of how dehydration can manifest itself will help prevent some migraines before they start. Here are the possible signs:

1. Mild Dehydration
2. Dry mouth or throat
3. Fatigue, weakness
4. Mild headache
5. Dark-coloured urine
6. Dizziness
7. Moderate to Severe Dehydration
8. Intense thirst
9. Confusion
10. Rapid heartbeat
11. Severe headache or migraine
12. Muscle cramps
13. Fainting
14. Electrolyte Imbalance
15. Muscle weakness
16. Irregular heartbeat
17. Nausea
18. Dizziness or "brain fog.".

If these symptoms are occurring, especially when a migraine is beginning, then take action regarding your hydration and electrolyte balance right away.

PRACTICAL STEPS IN HYDRATION AND BALANCE OF ELECTROLYTES

1. Establish Your Hydration Target:

A good benchmark will be about 8 to 10 glasses of water a day, but it might be different or more depending on your physical build, your activities, and your environment.

Hydration Goal for Migraine Patients: Consider drinking a glass of water every hour or so, especially if you are active or live in a warm climate. This gradual intake can help keep hydration levels steady.

2. Drink Electrolyte-Rich Beverages

Electrolyte drinks are especially beneficial if you are active, sweating profusely, or showing signs of dehydration. If you suffer from migraines, you should use low-sugar or no-sugar available because high sugar levels may result in blood sugar spikes, which could lead to a headache.

Homemade Electrolyte Drinks:

Prepare your own electrolyte drink using water with a pinch of sea salt, a squeeze of lemon, and a touch of honey or coconut water for added potassium.

Coconut Water:

Coconut water is also an all-natural source of potassium and other electrolytes, so you can use that in its place as a sports drink.

3. Make Hydration Food

Besides drinking water, you can hydrate with hydration foods also. Hydrating foods are very important because they are not just hydrating but contain essential vitamins and minerals in your body. It can come in the form of watermelon, cucumber, oranges, or leafy greens.

Hydration foods: Snack on sliced cucumber, melons, or oranges when it is hot and during intense physical training. These foods hydrate your body and are gentle to your stomach.

4. Controlling Caffeine and Alcohol Intake

Caffeine and alcohol can be considered as diuretics, thereby increasing the quantity of urine that could result in dehydration from excessive intake.

Limit Caffeine: Although some caffeine can assist with migraines, consume this substance only in moderation and drink additional water along with it. One easy way to put this principle into action is to have an extra glass of water with each glass of caffeinated drink.

Drink Alcohol in Moderation: If you're going to consume alcohol, drink at a slow pace and alternate between glasses of water. Try to avoid drinking diuretic beverages like beer or wine, which have more diuretics in them.

5. Take Magnesium Supplement if Necessary

One of the major electrolytes for someone with migraine is magnesium. Use supplements of magnesium if your diet is magnesium-deficient from food sources or you suspect a deficiency. Be sure to discuss with your healthcare provider any supplements you are going to take.

High-Magnesium Foods: Incorporate these high magnesium content foods in your diet like spinach, pumpkin seeds, almonds, black beans, and avocados.

Magnesium: Some people who develop migraines report that supplementing magnesium- either as glycinate or citrate- helps alleviate their attacks. "Discuss a dosing schedule with your physician tailored just for you," the doctors continue.

6. Be Aware of Your Hydration Patterns

Use a reminder app for drinking water. Alternatively, set reminders on your phone. Drinking more water may allow you to become better attuned to your dehydration states-especially during busy times.

Keep a Hydration Journal: Calibrate your hydration level, food intake, and your migraine symptoms in a journal. As you do this over time, you can begin to see the patterns that will help optimise your hydration for migraine prevention.

HOW TO IMPLEMENT DAILY HYDRATION

Hydration and electrolyte balance can easily be one of the simplest aspects of your daily routine. Here's a simple plan to get started:

Morning: Rehydrate as soon as you wake, with a glass of water - replenish after your sleep. Add some sea salt if you like, a few pinches for added electrolytes.

During the day: Drink water at least once every hour. Snack on hydrating foods, such as cucumbers, berries or citrus fruits.

After Physical Activity: Rehydrate with water and low-sugar electrolyte drink if you are sweating and exercising.

Evenings: Avoid caffeine and alcohol in the evenings. The choice of a light herbal tea or water for bed is enough.

CONCLUSION

Drink adequate amounts of water when it's hot outside, when you are engaging in some form of exercise, or if you are experiencing migraine symptoms.

Balance electrolytes by consuming sufficient magnesium, potassium, calcium, and sodium through food and drinks.

Avoid diuretics like caffeine and alcohol as they may worsen dehydration.

Supplementing with magnesium can reduce the number of attacks and make them less severe. Ask your physician if it is appropriate for you.

In the following chapter, we proceed to talk about another important concern for migraine prevention is the role of sleep and stress management. Good sleep and proper response to stress are one of the two essential factors that influence lowering the frequency and severity of migraine attacks, and by understanding how these concerns alter the equation regarding migraines, you will be equipped with the necessary ability to improve lifestyle changes to work toward improving your overall health.

CHAPTER 9: THE IMPACT OF SLEEPING AND THE MANAGEMENT OF STRESS IN TREATING MIGRAINES

Migraines have been said to be "an illness of the nervous system." This can only happen because sleep and stress influence the central nervous system profoundly. Poor sleep and chronic stress can increase vulnerability to migraines, while restful sleep and effective management of stress can act as guards against it. Studies show that while migraines are triggered by stress, they are also exacerbated by sleep, and by addressing both, you may be able to actually see the reduction of your frequency and intensity of your migraines.

This chapter dives deeper into the science of sleep and stress as it relates to migraine, offering actionable techniques for improvement in both.

THE ROLE OF SLEEP IN MIGRAINE PREVENTION

The scientists agree that everyone needs sleep, but in migraine patients, it is essentially different. During a good night's sleep, the body recharges, restores energy levels, and balances and adjusts the chemicals of the brain which may be in response to pain. Now, here's how sleep affects migraines:

1. Hormonal Regulation

Since the body controls and manufactures hormones during deep sleep, like cortisol and melatonin; altered sleep would then lead to an imbalance in the levels of these hormones: when its levels are out of whack, people may feel sensitised to pain and stress, plus become more sensitive to the migraine triggers.

2. Serotonin and Neurotransmitters

Serotonin is the neurotransmitter that helps modulate the mood and the pain, and indeed is very much affected by sleep, because low serotonin triggers migraines, while abnormal sleep can disrupt the serotonin, raising the likelihood of having one.

3. Brain Detoxification

The brain cleans up during its sleep, removing metabolic wastes and toxins. Dysfunction of this "brain cleansing" might make a more inflammatory and a prone place for causes of migraines.

4. Pain Threshold

Without adequate rest, the pain threshold is diminished. The body will become ever more sensitive to minor pain stimuli and find it harder to cope with symptoms of migraine or even trigger an attack.

RELATIONSHIP BETWEEN STRESS AND MIGRAINES

Probably the most common migraine trigger is stress. Stress puts your body into a 'fight or flight' response, thus releasing stress hormones like cortisol and adrenaline. Chronic stress may lead to over-reactions of the nervous system in people who are predisposed to developing migraines. This is how stress can affect your migraines:

1. Tension and Muscle Tightness

Stress causes tension on muscles, particularly in the neck and shoulders, that would bring about headaches and migraine.

2. Hormonal Response

 The levels of hormones in the body are interfered with by stress, especially cortisol. This leads to the interruption of blood flow, inflammation, and sensitivity to pain. Eventually, this enhances the frequency and severity of a migraine attack.

3. Hyperarousal of the Nervous System

Stress does not abate; it is continuing, which means that the nervous system remains in a constant state of hyper-arousal. This alone can be the stimulus to start a migraine headache. Stress can be so roller-coaster like that it becomes an added cause of the migraines, and so on.

4. Maladaptive Coping

When people experience stress, they often resort to coping strategies. These can be over-reliance on caffeine or lousy eating habits that become other causative factors for the migraines.

STRATEGIES TO BETTER SLEEP

To get quality sleep, it is not merely about the quantity-it's a matter of building habits and ensuring that the sleep you get is restful, sleep-centre deep. Some strategies to improving sleep follow:

1. Be Consistent about a Sleep Schedule

If you go to bed and wake up at the same time each day, you will regularise your internal clock-your body's circadian rhythm. This increases the quality of sleep and helps you have easier restorative sleep cycles for your body.

Tip: Use an alarm to set not only when you want to wake up but also at what time you will be going to bed to remind you to wind down at the same time every night.

2. Create a Soothing Pre-Bed Routine

A bedtime routine signals the body that it is time to sleep and minimises pre-sleep stress and anxiety.

Calming activities include reading, listening to soothing music or relaxing in a warm bath, or doing gentle stretching or yoga. Keep away from screens because the effects of the blue light emanating from them interfere with melatonin production.

3. Avoid Caffeine and Alcohol

Caffeine and alcohol disrupt sleep patterns. Because caffeine is released in the system for many hours, the best option to improve the quality of sleep is avoiding it in the afternoon and evening. Alcohol, although at first, is a sedative, disrupts deep sleep cycles and leads to broken sleep.

4. Prepare Your Sleeping Conditions

All factors, for example room temperature, light, and noise, have to be controlled so you may have a comfortable rest. A dark, cool, and silent room has to be obtained for better sleep.

Tip: Blackout curtains, cool it up to about 60-67 °F for most people, and white noise machine if you are noise-sensitive.

5. Try Relaxation Techniques Before You Go to Bed

Meditation, deep breathing, and progressive muscle relaxation may help calm the mind and body and get ready to sleep.

Progressive Muscle Relaxation: You start by tensing and relaxing one muscle group at a time, from toes to head. This process might help you drain tension stored in the muscles because of stress.

6. Magnesium Supplements for Good Rest

Magnesium is said to be soothing to the body and can relax the muscles. It is widely used for improving sleep and, therefore reduces stress.

Suggested Supplement: Consult your physician if magnesium glycinate will suit your body. It is said to be gut-friendly.

STRESS MANAGEMENT ACTIVITIES TO PREVENT MIGRAINES

Stress is a major factor that can significantly contribute to the frequency and severity of migraine. You can prevent a good deal of migraines by learning how to manage stress. Here are some stress management activities:

1. Meditation and Mindfulness

Both mindfulness and meditation train one's brain to better cope with stressful moments in healthier ways. Studies also reveal that these can reduce stress, improve mood, and even reduce migraine frequency.

Guided Meditation Apps. Headspace, Calm, and Insight Timer are just some of the guided meditation apps which may be of greater utility for beginners.

2. Regular Physical Activity

One of the best ways to deal with stress and make oneself generally healthier is exercise. Exercise is a stimulator that brings endorphins, a natural stress reliever in the body, bringing higher moods and low stress levels.

Low Impact: Walking, swimming, or cycling are good activities for people with migraines because they offer stress relief without too much strain on the body.

3. Deep Breathing Exercises

Deep breathing helps activate the body's relaxation response, which lowers the heart rate and blood pressure, neutralising the stress.

Simple techniques like "4-7-8 breathing" can even have instant calming effects. 4-7-8 Breathing Technique is to breathe in through the nostrils for a count of 4. Hold the breath for a count of 7, then breathe out slowly through the mouth with a count of 8. Repeat this several times to calm the mind.

4. Journaling to Prevent Emotional Build-Up

Putting your thoughts, concerns, or feelings on paper can help blow off steam and make the constant stressors put in perspective. Keeping a regular journal can really be effective in helping you cope with stress and track your migraine triggers.

Gratitude Journal: Try writing down three things you are grateful for at the end of each day. This helps divert your attention from stress and promotes a more positive mindset.

5. Setting Boundaries and Taking Care of Yourself

Most people cannot say no, so burning and chronic stress can be quite common. Good boundaries for self-care must be set at work or with personal relationships, combined with regular self-care to help decrease stress.

Examples of Self-Care: Set some time aside at the end of the week to do something just for you - perhaps hobbies, nature, or just relaxation with a good book.

6. Consider Cognitive Behavioral Therapy (CBT)

The goal of CBT is to enable a patient to identify and change those pervasive thought patterns and behaviours that cause his or her stress. Research has shown that CBT can reduce migraine frequency and help improve coping strategies.

Find a CBT Therapist: Many therapists specialise in CBT for stress and anxiety, and some even do sessions virtually. It can give you the tools to handle your stress triggers, so it is highly helpful to those who get stress-induced migraines.

CONCLUSION

Try your best to go to bed and wake up at the same time each day, maintain a bedtime routine that relaxes you, and generally try to avoid more stimulants like caffeine and alcohol.Mindfulness, exercise, and relaxation techniques can reduce migraine triggers.

Experiment with different techniques, such as meditation, journaling, or therapy, that best work for you to deal with stress and help you sleep better.

The following chapter explains how regular exercise can prevent migraine attacks. We can consider these health benefits of exercise, such as stress relief, improved circulation, and regulation of hormones, to reduce the risk of migraine attacks in our lives

CHAPTER 10: EXERCISE AND PHYSICAL ACTIVITY IN PREVENTING MIGRAINE.

Exercise and Physical Activity in Preventing Migraine For many, physical exercise is a panacea when it comes to health and wellness, but a double-edged sword for those who experience migraine. Exercise reduces stress and improves mood and circulation-all of which contribute to reducing the risk of migraine. However, for many, stressful or intense exercise can be a trigger, particularly if the body is not well-prepared or hydrated. This chapter will help you understand how to introduce exercise safely into your lifestyle as well as what types of activities may be most useful, along with some specific tips that will avoid exercise-induced migraines.

BENEFITS OF EXERCISE TO MIGRAINE SUFFERERS

Exercise positively affects the body and the brain in a number of ways that may help decrease the number and severity of migraines:

1. Increased Blood Circulation and Oxygenation

Exercise ensures the proper functioning of blood circulation in all parts of the body, including the head, thus oxygenating more body cells. Better circulation can prevent the vascular problems that are the cause of a migraine: narrowed or constricted blood vessels.

2. Hormone Regulation

One of the ways in which physical activity regulates hormones that control mood and pain perception is by balancing chemicals such as endorphins and serotonin, giving exercise a chance to prevent hormonal ups and downs that might stimulate a migraine.

3. Low Stress and Anxiety

Exercise is arguably one of the finest stress-relieving and anxiety-reducing behaviours. Regular physical activity has been shown to decrease levels of cortisol, the stress hormone, which is a known migraine trigger.

4. Improve Your Quality of Sleep

Exercise is also linked with improved quality of sleep that is an essential migraine prevention factor since one of the types of migraine headaches usually begins with feelings of extreme tiredness. Exercise will increase the amount of deep, restorative sleep one gets which keeps fatigue at bay.

5. Weight Management

For other people, weight gain or obesity might cause the risk for migraines. Regular exercise and other physical activity could support the upholding of the appropriate weight, reducing attacks' frequency.

EXERCISE AS A MIGRAINE TRIGGER: WHAT YOU NEED TO KNOW

While exercise offers so many benefits, some people do find that intense physical activity can trigger migraines. This is more commonly referred to as "exercise-induced migraines." These headaches may come on at the time of strenuous activities or after such activities and can occur if proper hydration, warm-up, or recovery practices aren't followed.

CONTRIBUTING FACTORS TO EXERCISE-INDUCED MIGRAINES

Dehydration: Because the body is not able to perform at its best, it illustrates headache symptoms when it is not hydrated enough.

Low Blood Sugar: Exercise during fasting or when the blood sugar levels are low can lead to a migraine.

Intense Activity: Sudden, very intense bursts of activity, such as sprinting or heavy weightlifting, suddenly puts a demand on the cardiovascular system, and this may trigger migraines.

If you're an exercise-induced migraine sufferer, try sticking with moderate steady activities, and take preventive measures to make exercise more comfortable and migraine-friendly.

BEST EXERCISES TO PREVENT MIGRAINES

A moderate, regular activity routine can be helpful, not high-intensity exercise for a person experiencing migraines. Among the best exercise types are:

1. Low-Impact Aerobics

Low-impact aerobic activities include walking, cycling, and swimming. Their intensity increases gradually without much pressure on the body system. They improve blood circulation, promote endorphin release, which reduces pain sensitivities.

Walking is an excellent activity since a brisk walk outdoors can help alleviate stress, as well as maximise one's mood and relax it at the same time.

Swimming is a low-impact, full-body exercise that requires less wear and tear on bones and joints. This can be highly beneficial for anyone who carries tension or stress-related migraines.

2. Yoga and Stretching

Yoga, by itself, is very useful in preventing such migraines, as the practice yields both physical movement and breathing and relaxation techniques. In fact, most suffering people are known to have found relief in practising yoga, as this practice has been known to reduce tension, lower stress, and also improve flexibility.

Relaxing Yoga Poses to Relieve a Headache such as Child's Pose, Forward Fold, and Legs Up the Wall are all very relaxing poses in which one can let go of tension in the muscles of the neck and shoulders, which are so often over-activated regions during a migraine headache.

Breathwork/Meditation such as many yoga classes involve deep breathing or meditation practice. These practices have been understood to actually activate the relaxation response in the body and to decrease the levels of stress.

3. Pilates and Core Strengthening

It focuses its movements on control and cultivates strength around the core. It improves people's posture and reduces neck and back pains. Working in these areas can help reduce migraine causes such as muscle tension and poor posture.

4. Tai Chi and Qigong

Tai Chi and Qigong are ancient Chinese exercises that connect gentle, flowing movements with mindful breathing. These exercises can help to calm the nervous system, reduce stress, and prevent loss of balance-all three of which are wonderful factors in helping to control a migraine.

Mind-Body Connection by Tai Chi and Qigong also link the body to the mind that can contribute to relaxation, particularly for those whose migraines are stress-related.

5. Strength Training (with Caution)

Moderate strength training can condition the muscles and enhance posture, and the patient must start from simple steps and exclude acute impacts. Great demands should be shown on the lighter weight and controlled movement. Therefore, many people note that heavy lifting sometimes causes them migraines.

TIPS FOR AVOIDING EXERCISE-INDUCED MIGRAINES

Here are some helpful strategies to enjoy the benefits of exercise without triggering migraines.

1. Stay Hydrated

Drink enough water before, during, and after exercising. Proper hydration helps prevent dehydration, which is one of the most common migraine triggers. Hydrate before, during, and after the workout session. Drink sufficient water throughout the day, especially when you have outdoor or warm workout sessions.

Electrolytes: When exercising longer periods, you might take an electrolyte drink with a low sugar content to restock the sodium, potassium, and other essential minerals lost through sweat.

2. Fuel Up Before Exercise

Low blood sugar can induce migraines, so you always want to have a light snack before exercising, certainly if you haven't eaten lately. For the greatest gains and productivity, consider a complex carbohydrate combined with protein.

Snack Ideas: A small banana with almond butter, yoghurt with berries, or a handful of nuts will provide quick energy without spiking blood sugar.

3. Warm Up and Cool Down

Intensities of exercise often have an immediate impact upon the cardiovascular system if warming up does not occur, and in fact, is one of the most common triggers for a migraine. A proper warm-up prepares the body for exercise, whereas a cool-down prevents the heart rate from suddenly falling.

Warm-Up Exercises: Use 5–10 minutes of light aerobic activity, which can be as simple as walking or gentle stretching.

Cool-Down Routine: End your exercise session by slowing down your movements and finishing with smooth stretches that also can relax muscles and relieve tension.

4. The Steadiness is the winner

In terms of migraine prevention, consistency beats intensity. Exercise as regularly as you are able to but at a pace that is comfortable for you. Do not overexert yourself and listen to what your body says; over-exercising can bring about the exercise headaches as well.

5. Learn to Breathe

The focus should be intense, deep, and slow breathing during exercises. It is more than likely to calm down the nervous system without building up stress. This proves particularly useful in reducing tension and stress-induced migraines.

Deep Breathing at Exercise: Slowly take deep breaths through the nose, filling the lungs to capacity and then exhaling completely. Such breathing helps defend against hyperventilation, sometimes causing headache.

6. Gradually Increase Exercise Intensity

Gradually build intensity if it's been a while since you exercise or if you just recently started exercising. Start slow and low impact. You should expect your body to gradually adapt, and may even let you do things that are a little tougher than what you're doing already.

Slow Start: Begin with 10-20 minutes of activity and then gradually add 5-10 minutes as your endurance goes up.

DEVELOP A PATTERN FOR ONGOING EXERCISE

Some of the lifestyle modifications that may make the most difference in treating migraines are creating an exercise routine. Here's an example week workout schedule:

1. Monday

Activity: 30 minutes brisk walk

Focus: Aerobic exercise to enhance blood circulation and evoke endorphins

2. Tuesday- Rest

3. Wednesday

Activity: Yoga session for 45 minutes

Focus: Flexibility improvement and relaxation enhancement

4. Thursday: Rest

5. Friday

Activity: 30 minutes Pilates or core exercises

Focus: Strengthening of the core muscles and muscle relaxation

6. Saturday: Rest

7. Sunday

Activity: 20 minutes of Tai Chi or Qigong

Focus: Mind and body connect for relaxation

This plan provides a combination of low-impact aerobics, strength, and relaxation activities that will prevent the migraine without overexertion.

CONCLUSION

Exercise for Prevention: Regular moderate exercise improves blood flow, manages stress, and balances hormone levels, which all decreases the migraine frequency.

Low-Impact Aerobic Activities such as Tai Chi and mind-body exercises are low-impact aerobic activities that help encourage gentle ease with a decrease in physical tension.

Listen to Your Body like Avoid overexertion and pace activities to what you know feels comfortable. Hydrate, fuel up, and look to increase intensity.

In the next chapter we will discuss dieting Strategies for Migraine Prevention.

CHAPTER 11 NUTRITION AND DIET APPROACHES TO PREVENTING MIGRAINES

Diet is a very effective tool in the management of migraines. For some, particular foods or ingredients will be triggers for migraine attacks, while in others, a deficiency in certain nutrients predisposes to attacks. You can, therefore, understand how your food intake - including that which you choose to avoid - affects the development of migraines and then create a diet that minimises triggers, reduces inflammation, and supports overall brain health.

THE CONNECTION BETWEEN DIET AND MIGRAINES

Basically, food is fuel for the body, and what you eat, drink, or don't do influences your mood, cognition, and general function. However, in a migraineur, the right foods and patterns of eating can be particularly influential. Here's how diet impacts migraines:

1. Blood Sugar Levels

Spiking and crashing in blood sugar can initiate a migraine. Balanced meals with complex carbohydrates, protein, and healthy fats may help your body maintain blood sugar levels without shocking them up or down.

2. Inflammation

Some foods, mostly processed and sugary products, trigger inflammation, which is strongly related to migraine. Antioxidant/anti-inflammatory foods such as fruits, vegetables, and healthy fats will contribute to lowering inflammation to prevent the onset of disease.

3. Lack of Nutrients

Lack of some nutrients, such as magnesium, riboflavin, or vitamin B2, and coenzyme Q10, has been associated with an increased risk for migraine attacks. Adding these nutrients to your diet or supplementing them may help.

4. Trigger Foods

Some foods contain natural substances that act as common triggers for people with migraines. These include tyramine, caffeine, and histamine. Determine your real individual trigger and keep your life free of those things.

FOODS THAT HELP RELIEVE MIGRAINES

There are foods that could supply anti-inflammatory, stabilising properties, and brain-boosting effects. Here's the best type of food to add your migraine-preventive diet:

1. Leafy Green Veggies

Leafy greens, including spinach, kale, and Swiss chard, are rich in magnesium-an essential nutrient for relaxing muscles, aiding nerve function and regulating blood pressure. Thus, these have been promoted through studies claiming people with low levels of magnesium tend to experience migraines.

2. Fatty Fish

Other than the elaboration of the guidelines, omega-3 fatty acids coming from foods such as salmon, sardines, and mackerel prevent inflammation and enhance neurological functions. Because omega-3 inhibits inflammation, it heals cardiovascular health and reduces migraine onsets, which may limit such adverse events because of the balanced level of inflammation and better cardiovascular system.

3. Whole Grains

Whole grains and its products, such as oats, quinoa, and brown rice, contain complex carbohydrates that stabilise blood sugar levels. This is deemed crucial in preventing dips of blood sugar that may send the subject to experience migraine signs and symptoms.

4. Nuts and Seeds

Almonds, sunflower seeds, and chia seeds contain a good amount of magnesium that is an absolute necessity for nerve health. All these snacks are easy to carry with you and can be easily added to your meals; they help prevent hunger migraine.

5. Hydrating Foods

Although excellent hydrators, cucumbers, watermelon, and celery have extremely high water content, which will help resolve dehydration-related migraines. Probably one of the key conditions for the migraine sufferer is good hydration; nothing better than water-rich foods to complement this.

6. Fresh fruits and berries

Fruits such as apples, pears, and blueberries are rich in antioxidants, have anti-inflammatory properties, and provide natural sugars for a steady flow of energy without causing a rapid rise or fall of blood sugar.

7. Lean Protein

Lean protein sources include chicken, turkey, and tofu, all of which stabilise blood sugar while helping to produce energy. If a person eats protein at every meal, they are likely to be much less hungry, and blood sugars will level out better, greatly decreasing their chances for migraines.

NUTRIENTS PROVEN TO TREAT MIGRAINES

There are some nutrients, however, known to prevent migraines. If you tend to have migraines, try and get these in your diet or talk with your healthcare provider about supplements:

1. Magnesium

Magnesium controls nerve functioning as it also reduces spasm and blood pressure. Foods rich in magnesium are spinach, pumpkin seeds, and black beans.

2. Riboflavin or B2

Another nutritional supplement that has been shown to reduce the rate of migraines is Vitamin B2. Foods that are good sources of this include eggs, dairy products, lean meats, and almonds.

3. Coenzyme Q10 (CoQ10)

CoQ10 is an antioxidant that relates directly to a healthy functioning of mitochondria and energy production. Foods that contain coenzyme Q10 are beef, chicken, and fatty fish, though it may be easier to take it as a supplement for migraine prevention.

4. Omega-3 Fatty Acids

These fatty acids, found in fish and flaxseeds, have intense anti-inflammatory effects. Omega-3 helps reduce inflammation in the brain and promotes cardiovascular health, which are factors that migraineurs need to have.

FOODS TO AVOID FOR MIGRAINE PREVENTION

While food can sometimes act as an ally, there are others known to commonly trigger migraines. Identifying what these specific triggers are for you is key, but here are some of the most commonly mentioned food culprits:

1. Caffeine

In some individuals, caffeine may partially relieve the migraine itself, but overuse or withdrawal from it may trigger an attack. Limit intake and observe consistent rather than high fluctuating levels.

2. Alcohol

Red wine and beer, in particular, contain histamine and sulfites that may induce an attack. If alcohol is a trigger, reduce it to the lowest amount possible or avoid it altogether.

3. Aged Cheeses

A good example is that cheddar, blue cheese, and parmesan contain a very high amount of tyramine, which is known to induce a migraine in many people.

4. Processed Meats

Hot dogs, sausages, and all other processed meats contain nitrates and nitrites. Both cause the blood vessels to dilate, or widen, which often brings in a migraine in sensitive people.

5. MSG and Artificial Additives

MSG, as a frequent flavour enhancer, and other unnatural preservatives may cause severe migraine headaches. Food items from packaging and fast foods are preferably to be avoided and replaced by fresh natural ingredients.

6. Chocolate

Chocolate contains caffeine and tyramine. Therefore, chocolate could be a trigger for those who suffer from migraines. If chocolate has been identified as a trigger, it is best to avoid it altogether or opt for carob.

CREATING A BALANCED MIGRAINE-PROMISING DIET

Balance, variety, and awareness are the fundamentals of creating a migraine-friendly diet. Here are some tips to get started:

1. Eat Consistently

Eat regular meals and snacks throughout the day to keep blood sugar levels steady. Avoid going long stretches without eating as this causes spikes and dips in blood sugar, a frequent migraine trigger.

2. Choose Whole, Unprocessed Foods

Whole foods are vegetables, fruits, whole grains, lean proteins, and healthy fats. They are so nutrient-rich, devoid of added preservatives, additives, or artificial ingredients that can activate a migraine.

3. Track Your Triggers

Maintaining a food diary can sometimes help you see what foods and ingredients are causing your migraines. Food diary tracking may show you which meals to be more conscious of with these problematic foods and ingredients.

4. Emphasise Anti-Inflammatory Foods

Opt for anti-inflammatory foods by selecting more whole fruits, vegetables, and whole grains combined with lean proteins and healthy fats.

Add a lot of anti-inflammatory foods to your diet, such as berries, leafy greens, and omega-3-rich foods, to help decrease inflammation in your body as well as to help feed your brain.

5. Supplement

Supplements are sometimes necessary where dietary intake alone is not feasible. Common migraine prevention supplements include magnesium, riboflavin, and CoQ10.

6. Hydrate

Drink plenty of water throughout the day because dehydration is the most common migraine cause. Aim to consume at least eight glasses of water daily, but this will increase if you are physically active.

MIGRAINE-FRIENDLY MEAL PLAN

Here's a sample day of migraine-friendly meals incorporating key nutrients and excluding known triggers.

Breakfast

Spinach and avocado smoothie made with almond milk, chia seeds, and one banana

Lunch

Quinoa salad with mixed greens, grilled chicken, cucumbers, and a lemon-tahini dressing.

Snack

A serving of blueberries and almonds Or Apple slices with almond butter

Dinner

Baked salmon with roasted sweet potatoes and steamed broccoli

CONCLUSION

Eat Frequently because regular meals maintain stable blood sugar levels, thus lowering the risk for migraines. Incorporate Anti-Inflammatory Foods because Leafy greens, fatty fish, berries, and nuts reduce inflammation and promote neuronal health. Keep a log of your eating and your experiences to identify what might be triggering your migraines through caffeine, alcohol, or certain processed meats.

Use these strategies to construct an eating plan that nourishes you while helping you to avoid things that could trigger migraines. In the following pages, we will examine the supplementation and alternative therapies to treat migraine and other, non-invasive options.

CHAPTER 12: SUPPLEMENTS AND COMPLEMENTARY THERAPIES FOR THE RELIEF OF MIGRAINE

Complementary and alternative therapies offer a vital intervention strategy for patients with migraines for whom conventional therapies are not as effective or bear intolerable side effects. Fortunately, several natural supplements and alternative therapies have been found to be useful in migraine management. Ranging from vitamins and minerals to herbal remedies and hands-on therapies, these supplements and complementary therapies could provide valuable additions to a migraine-prevention plan.

WHY SUPPLEMENTS AND ALTERNATIVE TREATMENTS?

Management of migraines can be holistic. In addition to diet, hydration, and sleep forming the cornerstone, some of the nutritional deficiencies can be plugged by targeted supplements, while alternative therapies can provide additional support that is sometimes drug-free. Here are the ways in which supplements and alternative treatments help:

1. Addressing Nutritional Deficiencies

The most commonly deficient nutrients are magnesium and vitamin B2, and lesser-known CoQ10. You will be protecting yourself from getting a migraine, before it has occurred, by supplementing your body with the aforementioned nutrients.

3. Relaxing Muscle Tension

There are other therapies that can help relax muscles-possibly through acupuncture or massage-which also could help move a migraine along. Tensing up of muscles is indeed a common cause of migraine pain, though the pain is most closely associated with it in migraine patients who also suffer from tension-type headaches.

GOOD PREVENTIVE SUPPLEMENTS FOR MIGRAINES

Many supplements have been studied for their efficacy in preventing migraine headaches. Here are some of the most promising among these supplements:

1. Magnesium

Magnesium is an important mineral for nervous system function, although it has a crucial role in regulating neurotransmitters and preventing nerve overactivity, which might actually cause migraines. The results of studies indicate that the patients with migraine have a lower magnesium concentration than healthy individuals. Supplementation may decrease both frequency and intensity of attacks.

Recommended Dosage: Take 400-500 mg per day as magnesium citrate or magnesium glycinate for easier absorption and fewer gastrointestinal side effects.

Apart from these, magnesium enhances quality sleep while also eliminating anxiety and spasms within the muscles, all of which go to assist patients suffering from migraine attacks.

2. Riboflavin (Vitamin B2)

Vitamin B2, otherwise known as riboflavin, ensures proper cellular energy production, along with proper maintenance in functions for the brain. Low levels of riboflavin have been shown to be associated with a higher risk of suffering from migraine, and supplementing it has been seen to lessen the number of migraines a patient suffers from.

Dosage: 400 mg to be taken every day.

Other Benefits: B2 also supports the body in maintaining healthy skin in addition to supporting the eyes; there are further additional benefits for a healthy general wellness.

3. Coenzyme Q10 (CoQ10)

CoQ10 is an antioxidant at the cellular level, and it assists the body in providing energy, especially to the brain. Several studies have shown that supplementation with CoQ10 has decreased both frequency and severity of migraine attacks.

Dosage: 100–300 mg daily

Secondary Benefits: CoQ10 is beneficial to heart health, and this may particularly benefit those with migraines related to vascular problems.

4. Feverfew

Feverfew is an herbal remedy that has long been used to ward off migraines. It contains chemical constituents that prevent inflammation and might be able to prevent constriction of the blood vessels, which is often associated with a migraine.

Dosage Recommended : 100–300 mg per day (standardised for 0.2%–0.4% parthenolide)

Secondary Benefits: The herb may also have other secondary benefits to symptoms such as nausea and photosensitivity.

5. Butterbur

Anti-inflammatory herb used preventively to treat migraines. It is thought to act by reducing muscular spasms and inflammation that occur in association with migraine.

Dosage : 50–75 mg twice daily; remember to take a PA-free, standardised extract.

Additional value: Butterbur may also lessen the recurrence of allergy-type symptoms and thus is of utility·in patients with seasonal allergies.

Vitamin D

Low levels of vitamin D have been linked to migraine in patients who suffer frequent headaches. Vitamin D supplementation may, therefore help better control the inflammation and prevent episodes of attacks, especially in patients with previously diagnosed deficiency.

Dosage: 1,000–2,000 IU/day. Suspected deficiency: advise see doctor.

Other benefits: Vitamin D regulates immune systems and bone strength.

ALTERNATIVE THERAPIES FOR MIGRAINE MANAGEMENT

While supplements may be helpful, combining them with alternative treatments may actually double their effectiveness to provide medication-free relief. Some of the best alternative therapies for migraine prevention and relief include the following:

1. Acupuncture

It is a traditional Chinese practice of medicine wherein thin needles are introduced in the body at appropriate points. Researchers have proven how effective acupuncture is because it decreases, first of all, the rate of migraine occurrences and, secondly, the severity through helping its patients release their endorphin and inducing relaxation.

How it Helps: Acupuncture battles common migraine causes, like stress, muscle tension, or imbalances in the energy flow.

Considerations: Sessions are usually held once or twice a week in the early stages, which may decrease over time as the patient starts showing improvements.

2. Biofeedback

Biofeedback is a type of training that teaches control over physiological responses such as muscle tension and heart rate through guided relaxation and feedback. It's extremely helpful for stress-induced migraines and tension-type headaches.

How it Works: Biofeedback trains to prevent the onset of migraines by learning control over stress responses.

Considerations: This treatment is time-consuming because one has to acquire techniques over several sessions with an experienced therapist.

3. Cognitive Behavioural Therapy

CBT is a form of psychotherapy that aims to treat destructive lines of thinking that can lead to a stressful condition and physiological effects such as migraine. Some studies indicate it may decrease the number of attacks by dealing with stress and anxiety.

How It Helps: CBT targets the emotional aspects of migraines, which decreases stress and can lead to healthier coping practices.

Considerations: Ideally, meeting with a licensed therapist will prove most beneficial. CBT typically requires weeks or months of scheduled treatment.

4. Massage Therapy

Massage can relax tense muscles, improve circulation, and reduce stress—all beneficial in migraine management, particularly if the migraine is mediated at least in part by tension in the neck, shoulders, or back.

How It Helps: Massage relaxes knotted muscles, boosts blood flow, and releases endorphins; migraines occur less often

Considerations: More frequent massage sessions are required, but especially if your migraines tend to correspond with physical tension or poor posture.

5. Essential Oils and Aromatherapy

Some essential oils such as peppermint oil and lavender oil have been known to cause the release of a calming and pain-reducing effect. Aromatherapy can be very effective in treating migraines, especially when applied to address the early stages of a headache.

How It Helps: Peppermint oil applied on the temples can help ease tension headache, while lavender oil might reduce stress and promote relaxation.

Considerations: Essential oils should be used with caution as robust smells might sometimes make a migraine worse. Apply oils to a small area before using them to avoid irritation to the skin.

6. Cold and Warm Compresses

Cold compress on the forehead or heat compress to the neck helps to combat migraines as it relaxes tension in muscles and numbs the pain.

It works as cold therapy deadens pain or inhibits it and involves vasoconstriction in contracture of blood vessels that reduces the impact of the migraine, while applying heat to the neck deals with relaxing muscles and dilating blood vessels.

Considerations: Do compresses as soon as symptoms start to provide maximum relief. Alternating cold and warm compresses may also help.

SAFETY AND PRECAUTIONS

When Using Supplements and Alternative Therapies

Natural remedy treatments can be effective, but such remedies don't come without risks. Here are important precautions when you use these remedies safely:

1. Consult a Healthcare Provider

Before taking a new supplement or other alternative therapy-particularly if you are already on medication-be sure to consult your doctor first to ensure that it will not interact with your existing medication.

2. Gradual Intake

The introduction of a new supplement or therapy should begin with the lowest recommended dose or frequency to gauge your body's reaction to it.

3. Consistency

Natural remedies may take weeks to start working. Do not lose hope if you are not experiencing relief within a week. It sometimes takes at least a few weeks for someone to establish whether a supplement or therapy is working.

4. Follow Your Headaches

Keep a headache diary to figure out if any supplement or treatment is doing anything good for your headaches. Follow changes in frequency, severity, and triggers over time.

5. Choose Quality Products

Supplements: Use the highest-quality brand you can afford and standardised extracts of herbal supplements, such as feverfew and butterbur. Alternative therapies: Use only certified practitioners.

CONCLUSION

Typically deficient in people with migraine headaches are nutrients that include magnesium, riboflavin, and CoQ10; all have been shown to reduce attacks when supplemented.

Techniques that include acupuncture, biofeedback, and massage all help to relieve stress and tension, two major contributors to migraine.

Triggers are a bit different for everyone, so monitor the response to new supplements or treatments and adjust accordingly.

Supplements and Alternative Therapies can be an extremely effective natural supporter of managing migraines. In Chapter 13 we will explore environmental issues and how to minimise triggers in your environment-from lighting and noise to chemicals.

CHAPTER 13: MINIMISE ENVIRONMENTAL TRIGGERS TO STOP MIGRAINES

Environmental triggers for migraines are the most common. Lighting, noise, and air can induce headaches in sensitive people who cannot tolerate sensory stimuli. A migraine-friendly environment can greatly reduce the chances of an attack, thus making your surroundings the elementary part of migraine prevention.

In this chapter, we discuss the common environmental precipitants of migraines and some practical measures you can do to minimise their impact. Simple adjustments in your home, workplace, and daily lifestyle can really make a huge difference in migraine management.

COMMON ENVIRONMENTAL TRIGGERS

For someone who suffers with migraines, it's overwhelming when seemingly ordinary things become triggers for a migraine attack. Here are the most common environmental factors that may lead to a migraine attack:

1. Lighting and Glare Bright, flickering, or fluorescent lights can trigger migraines, but long periods of viewing the computer or other screen can as well. Sensitivity to light, or photophobia, is a common complaint of those who suffer from migraines and makes extremely bright places unbearable.

2. Noise and Sound Loud or penetrating noises, including construction, traffic, and even just crowded places, can sometimes stimulate headaches. Many headache patients have phonophobia, so minimising sound levels, where feasible, may be helpful.

3. Air Quality and Odours Poor quality of air, which also includes some strong smells of cleaning agents, perfumes, and chemicals, often triggers migraines. Osmophobia or sensitivity to smells is reported by most migraine patients; therefore, it is very important to control the smell and air quality.

4. Temperature changes or Humidity Sudden changes in temperature, too much heat, or very high humidity can be a trigger. Sometimes individuals suffer more from migraines in specific seasons or due to particular weather patterns.

5. Exposure to long periods of screen time-from the computer, tablet, or smartphone-results in exposure to blue light, a potential contributor to eye strain and migraine attacks.

6. Allergens: Seasonal allergens-pollen, mould, and dust-can trigger symptoms in some headache patients. Indoor allergens are also important, including dog and cat dander.

TAKING ACTIONS THAT MINIMISE EXPOSURE

Taking actions that minimise exposure to such triggers in your environment can really make a big difference in the management of your migraines.

1. Control Lighting

Use Natural Sunlight: Make use of natural sunlight when possible. This can easily be obtained if one uses soft, indirect sunlight instead of overhead lights which are most probably going to trigger a migraine.

Make a selection of Gently bulbs: Warm, low and dimmable LED or incandescent bulbs are much less likely to flicker or create harsh glare. Avoid fluorescent lighting, which may often flicker at frequencies that can trigger migraines.

Polarised Sunglasses: In fact, for individuals who experience migraines from bright lights or glare, using polarised sunglasses indoors, as well as outdoors can cut down eye strain and block out harmful rays.

You can install dimmer switches: Dimmer switches allow you to adjust the lighting by dimming, allowing you to turn down the brightness of light if it is too bright and help you to build a comfortable environment.

You can use Blue Light Glasses: If you regularly make use of your computer or mobile phone, taking precautions to minimise blue light emissions from screens help reduce chances of ending up with migraines from permanent exposure to the screens.

2. Controls Noise:

Use Earplugs or Noise-Cancelling Headphones: If you easily get disturbed by noise, earplugs or noise-cancelling headphones can help muffle the environment, especially in noisy public spaces or at work.

Create Quiet Zones: A quiet space in your house where one can withdraw for rest and solitude when cases of very noisy households apply.

Use White Noise Machines: White noise machines will mask sound interference, and help people relax and sleep easily even in noisy environments.

Minimise background noises: Avoid noise-causing machines like a television or loud music when working or sleeping. A quiet house is one big thing to help cut down on stress and migraines.

3. Improve Air Quality

Get an air purifier: An air purifier with HEPA filters eliminates most allergens, dust, and other unnoticeable pollutants in the air, giving you fresher air that can be beneficial in reducing headache triggers.

Avoid Strong Smells: Use fragrance-free or naturally fragranced cleaners and avoid perfume and scented candles. You can use essential oils, but some of those will work as a trigger too, so be cautious.

Ventilate Often: Open windows to let fresh air inside, diluting indoor pollution. Good airflow can help clear out cooking fumes, dust, and other irritants.

Make Use of Plants in Purifying the Air: Snake plants, peace lilies, and spider plants are some of the most popular houseplants that assist in clearing the air and producing oxygen.

4. Temperature Control and Humidity

Maintain a Comfortable Indoor Climate for Migraines: Maintain your dwelling at a relatively comfortable temperature for migraines. Do not overheat it, especially when you are sensitive to heat.

Humidifiers or Dehumidifiers: For dry climate persons, using humidifiers to raise moisture levels in the air is ideal, while persons staying in humid climates can make use of the dehumidifier to eliminate excess moisture from the air.

Wear Layers: Wearing layers allows one to easily change from one layer to another depending on the temperature around him/her, which may stop migraines resulting from hot or cold temperatures.

Avoid Direct Sun Exposure: If the sun's heat triggers migraines, limit exposure during hot times and spend more time in shaded or air-conditioned places as much as possible.

5. Limit Screen Exposure/Blue Light Exposure

Apply 20-20-20: Every 20 minutes take a 20-second break and look 20 feet away. This avoids the eyes getting too strained and perhaps even making it work for too long without a break to which it might trigger a migraine.

Adjust Your Screen Settings: Go to night mode or try setting your screen brightness at its lowest to decrease emission of blue light.

Set Blue Light-Free Times: Set times as blue light-free, especially before bed time. High exposure can interfere with sleep and trigger migraines.

Check for Apps that Block Blue Light: Most devices can access apps or settings that will reduce the emission of blue light. These are really helpful in the evening time when you're more prone to staying indoors.

6. Controlling Allergens and Reducing Triggers at Home

Keep your house clean. Dust and vacuum often. If you have a pet or pollen is rampant in your area, this will cut down on the allergens.

Beddings with hypoallergenic properties. Hypoallergenic beddings are meant to be the best options for those who have issues with dust mites allergy. Most of them are made of hypoallergenic materials to reduce allergy-related migraines.

Regularly wash linens. Dust and allergen accumulation of bed linens and curtains may pile up over time and cause migraine.

An HVAC Filter: Good quality air filters for the HVAC can reduce the indoor allergen load, thus overall improving indoor air quality.

Space that is inhospitable to a migraine may not only be free of egregious triggers, but also conducive to calm and relaxation. Here's how you make your space a restful sanctuary:

Designate your relaxation space: Designate a space where you always retreat to relax, meditate, or do whatever is comfortable in the moment. Even a room with soft lighting, comfortable seating, or perhaps books, blankets, or even plants can be what you need to soothe your senses.

Add a Natural Component: The evidence presumes that there is some soothing effect of nature. Incorporate as many plants or water features, or even the sounds of nature, in your space to make it calmer and less stressful, which is truly a migraine trigger.

Reduce Clutter: A cluttered space builds up stress. Ensure that your living environment is clean and free of clutter. This would make the space less overwhelming and support a more peaceful environment.

Incorporate soothing colours such as blues and greens with earth tones, which may not be more of a sensory overload.

CONCLUSION

Consider warm, indirect lighting over overhead fluorescents that may exacerbate light sensitivity.

Decrease Noise and Design quiet spaces and use noise-reduction headphones or earpieces that can minimise exposure to irritating noises and sounds.

Purify the air. Avoid pungent fragrances on clothes or uses, which can trigger a migraine from smells.

Keep the temperature in the house tolerable as well as control the humidity as necessary to avoid climate-induced triggers.

Observe the 20-20-20 rule as well as keep the brightness of monitors at a minimum to minimise digital eye strain.

Make your environment peaceful and organised, which is also a stress-reducing measure against migraine.

By regulating environmental triggers and ensuring a peaceful atmosphere, you will be able to minimise your risks of migraine in your surroundings. The next page will cover lifestyles and habits and routines that can further help you fight against your risks of migraine.

CHAPTER 14: LIFESTYLE HABITS FOR MIGRAINE PREVENTION

In addition to dietary changes and supplementations as well as environmental modification, lifestyle habits are an important consideration in the management of migraines. Like most of life, even those things over which we have no control can sway the severity or frequency of an attack. Lifestyle habits in terms of sleep, exercise, and tension, for example, can impact the frequency and the intensity of the migraine. Creating a habit of living that fosters stability and wellness can help your body to function better and, therefore, lower the probability of a migraine attack.

Included is an overview of lifestyle habits that might be supportive for migraine prevention, along with how-to tips on how to modify personal habits.

Why Lifestyle Matters in Migraine Management

Changes in routine or physical states of imbalance also cause migraines. Such imperfections include variations in the sleep-wake cycle, large amounts of stress, or inconsistent times for eating. Generally, a change in routine causes instability in the body, which may lead to a migraine condition. A balanced routine with good habits keeps the state stable, hence making the body firm enough to avoid attacks of migraines.

Good Habits of Migraine Lifestyle

1. Regular Sleep Schedule

Sleep is also one of the very important tools in the management of migraines. Poor sleep quality, inconsistent sleep patterns, or no rest could result in making the brain a bit more sensitive to triggers. Moreover, sleep deprivation is one of the prominent factors for migraine attacks.

Create a Sleep Routine: It is recommended that you sleep at approximately the same time of the day every night, whether it's a weekend or a weekday. Maintaining regular slumber patterns keeps your body's internal clock in balance and also enhances the quality of your sleep.

Create a Bedtime Ritual: Avoid any electronic or stimulating activities close to bedtime. Choose relaxing activities, such as reading a book, light stretches, or deep breathing exercises.

Limit Caffeine and Alcohol: Both caffeine and alcohol are stimulants. These can disrupt patterns if consumed close to bedtime. Limit intake and avoid these substances in the late afternoon and evening.

Maintain Your Bedroom Dark and Cool: Light and temperature play a big role in sleep quality. Maintain your bedroom dark, quiet, and cool for the most restful sleep.

2. Regular Physical Activity

Exercise is an excellent way to take control of the attacks because it can help you reduce stress, lift your mood, and maintain sleep. Other aerobic exercises like walking, swimming, and cycling can increase the level of endorphin and become natural pain relievers and mood stabilisers.

Choose Low-Impact Activities: Sometimes, high-impact activities can cause the migraines to trigger, especially during the onset. Therefore, start low-impact activities like walking, yoga, or swimming.

Regular Exercise: Be active for at least 30 minutes most days of the week. Consistency is key; one or two intense sessions will not generally prevent migraines, but regular moderate activity does.

Mindful Movement Yoga, tai chi, and Pilates: These are perfect to improve body awareness and to reduce tension by combining movement with mindfulness, calming your nervous system, and reducing levels of stress.

Keep Hydrated: Dehydration can be one of the exacerbating factors for migraines; especially on exercise days, drink water before, during, and after exercise.

3. Regular Eating Schedule and Balanced Nutrition

Discussed already in previous chapters, fluctuations in blood sugar is yet another common trigger. A balanced regular eating schedule ensures that there are no plunges and peaks of blood sugar drops which could lead to headaches.

Eat at Intervals: Avoid missing your meals; sometimes it resulted in hypoglycemia, which triggered the migraine. If possible, eat at fixed times to ensure stable release of energy into the body.

Eat Nutrient-Rich Foods: Focus on whole foods like vegetables, fruits, lean meats, and whole grains. These can be reliable sources of stable energy and good brain function.

Limit Sugary Foods and Processed Goods: Refined foods and sweet treats can create blood sugar spikes and crashes. Enjoy healthy options such as nuts, yoghurt, or fruit, if you need to be energised.

Hydration: Hydration is key. Enjoy a glass of water first thing in the morning and carry a bottle to remind you to drink regularly throughout the day.

4. Stress Management Methods

Stress is the most common migraine-triggering factor and learning to manage stress can take care of migraines so that their frequency may reduce.

Practice Mindfulness and Meditation: Mindfulness and meditation are ways in which a person learns how to be present, and to handle stress they are trying to minimise their migraines. Even 5 minutes of meditation in a day is crucial.

Deep Breathing Techniques: Diaphragmatic breathing, or deep belly breathing, will help calm the nervous system and release physical tension. It is an excellent way to reduce stress when used just a few times in stressful situations.

Learn to Say No and Avoid Overcommitting: Burnouts or overextensions often result from overcommitting or taking on too good of a thing. Learn to say "no," set rest periods, and allow yourself some time to decompress.

Explore Therapy: Consulting a therapist may prove helpful in dealing with tension, particularly in patients experiencing frequent migraine attacks. Among the therapies, cognitive behavioural therapy has been useful in the management of migraines because it helps alter thought patterns responsible for stress.

5. Reduction of Screen Time and Eye Care

A great factor that has been identified as a cause of migraines is digital screens, especially several hours of blue light exposure to the eyes that lead to a feeling of eye strain. High employment rates and hobby-related screen usage require the restriction of some screen time and good eye care for prevention.

Take Frequent Screen Breaks: Apply the 20-20-20 rule-view something 20 feet away for at least 20 seconds every 20 minutes. This will limit eye fatigue and keep you from spending too much time looking at screens.

Use Blue Light Filters: Most devices have a blue light filter or "night modes" that minimise exposure to blue light. Be sure to use these during the night.

Tweak your screens' brightness: Make the brightness comfortable to the eyes, and ensure that your screen is at your eye level, not below eye level, where you would be constantly forced to look up.

Avoid screens in bed: Overall, spending too much time on your screens before bed will disrupt sleep, so endeavour to keep those devices away from you at least an hour before your bedtime.

6. Healthy Social Routine

Social interactions and supportive networks decrease stress and emotional support-very important in migraine management.

Stay Connected: Being related to close people somehow turns out to be a buffer for stress. Find time to relate meaningfully with others, whether it's to friends, family, or groups with whom you can associate.

Join a Migraine Support Group: You can find some great online or local migraine support groups where you can get valuable advice and get meaningful emotional support from other people who know what you're going through. Nobody is alone; bringing your experiences forward with others can definitely make you feel less lonely in this situation.

Balance Social and Rest Time: More socialising will always be helpful, but too much of it at times may sometimes result in stress and fatigue, which are also triggers for migraines. Try to balance your social time with rest and self-care time.

Tips for Getting Them to Work

No one ever succeeds in changing everything at once. Here are some tips on how to navigate these lifestyle shifts:

1. Take it one habit at a time: Once you feel natural about it, add another. Small, consistent steps often prove more effective than large, sudden changes.

2. Set Achievable Goals In your diary: write a few achievable goals for example, drinking a certain amount of water glasses daily, or introducing one new meal to your weekly diet. Achievable goals minimise the chances of feeling overwhelmed.

3. Keeping a Track Record: Keeping track of the changes through the journal will help you to view the changes you have undergone over the period, and hence you will see the results of these changes in your migraines. Write what works well, and what should be adjusted.

4. Celebrate Small Wins: Acknowledge all of your efforts and improvements, no matter how small they are. Positive reinforcement may inspire you to just keep laying down healthy habits.

5. Be Patient With Yourself: It takes some time before new habits become ingrained. Don't forget that setbacks happen, and it's okay to be kind to yourself. Gradual steps are still steps in the right direction.

6. Maintain routines: Maintain regular sleep, eating schedules and frequency of exercise to reduce migraine frequency as all your body systems become stable.

7. Mindfulness and Relaxation: Stress is one main reason for inducing migraines. Reducing it by teaching mindfulness, breathing exercises, and keeping one's time correctly may prevent migraines.

8. Screen care and Eye care: Reduce eye strain with less screen time or even a break in between, using blue light filters to prevent screen-related migraines.

9. Social Support: The ability to sustain social relationships may alleviate stress because such relief is considered an essential resource in combating potential migraines.

CONCLUSION

These lifestyle habits, when developed habitually, thus offer a strong foundation in the prevention of migraines. Small daily alterations often lead to great long-term benefits, creating a stronger and more resilient lifestyle that resists migraine.

Finally, in the last chapter,we will walk you through summarising all-important takeaways from the book, distilling that into a comprehensive action plan, and empowering you on your journey toward headache-free living.

CHAPTER 15: PUTTING IT ALL TOGETHER-YOUR ACTION PLAN FOR HEADACHE-FREE LIVING

And so, after this guide has taken you through the final chapter, it's now time to put all of this together to form an actionable plan. Managing migraines involves diet change and alteration of lifestyle, changing the environment you are living in, or environments you will visit, including a proper relaxation or anti-stress strategy. The idea here is to give you realistic, science-based strategies that fit your life so you can more effectively prevent and alleviate migraine attacks.

Let's outline the basic steps within this chapter, and we'll build a fluid action plan that you can tailor for your needs. Remember that progress often takes time, and consistency is everything. So, let's get going on your individualised blueprint to headache-free living.

Step 1: Identify Your Triggers

Understanding what provokes your migraines is the first step to prevention. Migraines most often result from an interplay of several contributing factors, so every individual needs to know exactly what in their surroundings triggers theirs.

Keep a Migraine Diary: Write down each migraine you have in your diary or track it through an app. Note down any events occurring before the migraine, whether it's food consumption, stress levels, changes in sleep pattern, and changes in the environment around you. After a period of time, you will start to see repeating patterns that you can point to as culprits.

Identify Patterns: After a few weeks, look back over your entries to see if you can identify patterns. Are migraines associated with certain foods? Do they tend to occur at times of high stress? Determine these patterns so that you can modify your plan.

Step 2: Create an Anti-Migraine Diet

A healthy diet that is high in nutrients helps to reduce inflammation and will help control blood sugar that can trigger the migraine headache.

Get Rid of Known Triggers: Using observation, remove or lessen food that can cause your migraines. Caffeine and alcohol, processed foods, and additives are all common troublemakers.

Add Anti-Inflammatory Diets: Foods high in omega-3s, antioxidants, and fibre bring down inflammation. Take a look at the ways to add more salmon, leafy greens, turmeric, ginger, and berries to your diet.

Hydrate: Hydration is the secret, and you should make water your best friend. See to it that you drink at least 8 glasses of water a day and drink much more if you're active or you are exposed to hot temperatures.

Practise Balanced Eating: Do not starve yourself because skipping meals can lead to unstable blood sugar levels. It's therefore better to continue eating regularly by following specific times for each meal.

Step 3: Supplementation

While the bulk of the substance would come from a healthy diet, several supplements may add special support to preventing migraines. Each must be addressed with your health care provider before starting them.

Magnesium: Many people have lower levels than usual, and supplemental magnesium has been shown to decrease frequency of migraines. Include 200-400 mg per day and, in particular, magnesium glycinate or citrate because these are typically better tolerated by the digestive system.

Vitamin B2 (Riboflavin): Riboflavin may reduce the incidence of migraines in some patients. A supplement of 400 mg per day may be useful.

CoQ10: This antioxidant appears to support mitochondrial function and tends to be of benefit in lessening migraine headaches. Typical dosing has ranged between 100-300 mg per day.

Herbal Support: Two herbal preparations that are used in conventional practice to help control migraines are feverfew and butterbur. Be sure to use standardised supplements and only purchase this type of product from a reputable manufacturer so it is pure and safe.

Step 4: Have a Routine

Have routine habits every day. This will stabilise your body's internal clock and lower the chance of causing the migraine due to irregular habits.

Always ensure you have rest from 7-8 hours in a day, whereby bedtime and wake up hours are well consistent day in day out. Quality of sleep can be improved through a pre-sleep routine which is soothing.

Be Active Physically: Find time each week for regular, moderate exercise. Low-impact activities like walking and yoga, as well as swimming, tend to decrease stress without increasing migraines.

Eat Regular Meals: Maintain a consistent schedule for eating. Have some healthy snacks on hand to avoid low blood sugar.

Step 5: Learn to Manage Stress

Stress is the most common migraine trigger. By developing techniques to manage stress, you will begin to feel much better overall and notice your migraines are decreasing in frequency.

The stress-reducing activity of meditation and mindfulness helps keep the nervous system calm. Five to 10 minutes in a day can make all the difference in changing the way we react to stress.

Breathing Exercises: Fast control of tension can be achieved with deep breathing or diaphragmatic breathing. These techniques can be done during peak situations, helping to keep stress under control.

Delegate and Prioritise Self-Care: Effectual management of responsibilities, and even setting appropriate boundaries will keep you from getting overwhelmed. Self-care is your priority, such as taking time to do things that relax and rejuvenate you.

Step 6: Take Control of Your Environment

Earning control over your environment can sometimes keep the frequency and intensity of attacks at bay, especially among those sensitive to sensory triggers.

Use warm, indirect lighting with warm rather than bright fluorescents. If screens are an issue, use blue light filters and take regular breaks to cut eye strain.

Reduce Noise Exposure: Earplugs or noise-cancelling headphones can minimise sound-driven stress. Create a quiet space in your home to which you can retreat when you start to feel a headache strike.

Indoor Air Quality: Your migraines might be caused by reduced allergens and pollutants due to air purifiers. Avoid fragrances and use fragrance-free products or natural cleaning agents whenever possible.

Temperature and Humidity Control: For comfort, you can utilise fans, air conditioning, or humidifiers. Extreme temperatures and drastic changes in humidity may act as a trigger; therefore, it would make sense to maintain a controlled climate.

Day 7: Monitor Your Progress

Keeping track of your improvement will help you know which strategies are working best for you. Monitoring improvement can also keep you motivated to stay on the good habits.

Use a Migraine Tracker: Even now continue to track and monitor changes in frequency, intensity, or duration. This is how to evaluate which lifestyle changes are the most effective.

Celebrate Small Wins: Every improvement, no matter how small, brings us closer to better control over our migraines. Celebrate your wins to keep you positive and motivated.

Adjust as Needed: Your needs can change. Regularly review your routine and make adjustments for the time being to stay aligned with your body's needs.

CONCLUSION

Living migraine-free is a journey, and foremost, no one-size-fits-all solution. Rather, each of the strategies found in this book is an element of the jigsaw that fits together into a comprehensive scheme of prevention tailored to your lifestyle. Remember, the most successful strategy is the one you can sustain and adapt to your specific needs.

Being proactive and patient with changes in life is the key. Migraines can be very complicated and take a while to improve. Building supportive habits around nutrition, sleep, exercise, and stress management will create a foundation that supports your ongoing health and resilience. You will discover what works best for your life and be empowered to live it on your terms-free from migraine control of daily life.

That's it for the journey through Natural Migraine Relief. You now have a clear action plan and the tools to take control of your health and live life free from the burdens of headaches. Here's to a healthier, headache-free future!

Thank you